Researching the people's health

Researching the People's Health examines two related issues: the role of social research in the rapidly changing world of health services, and the relationship between lay and expert knowledge in public health and health care. The book examines these issues against the background of long-term transformations in patterns of health and illness, and rapid changes in the strategic management and commissioning of health services. In so doing the book makes a contribution to the continuing and urgent debates on the assessment of health needs, the organization and delivery of health care, and the politics of health services organization and funding.

Researching the People's Health is aimed at professionals and academics, and will be of particular interest to people working in public health, health promotion, health policy and the sociology of health and illness.

Jennie Popay is Professor of Community Health Studies at the University of Salford, and Director of the Public Health Research and Resource Centre, Bolton, Salford, Trafford and Wigan Health Authorities. **Gareth Williams** is Reader in the Sociology of Health and Illness in the Department of Sociology at the University of Salford.

Researching the people's health

Edited by Jennie Popay
and Gareth Williams

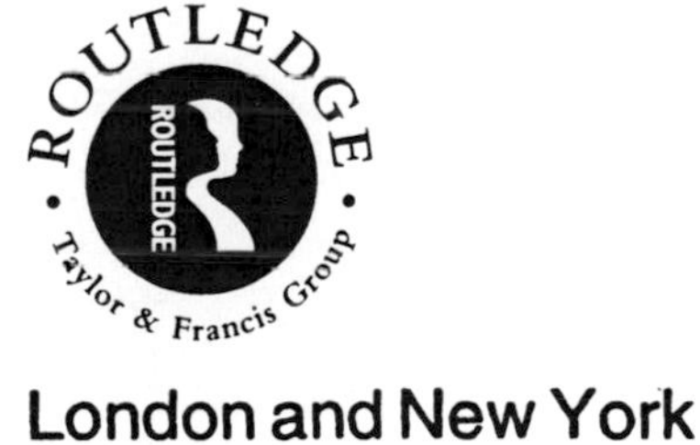

London and New York

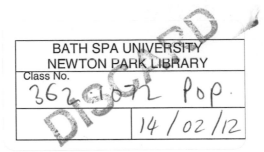

First published 1994
by Routledge
2 Park Square, Milton Park, Abingdon, Oxon, OX14 4RN

Simultaneously published in the USA and Canada
by Routledge
270 Madison Ave, New York NY 10016

Reprinted 2002

Transferred to Digital Printing 2005

Routledge is an imprint of the Taylor & Francis Group

Typeset in Times by LaserScript, Mitcham, Surrey

British Library Cataloguing in Publication Data
A catalogue record for this book is available from the British Library

Library of Congress Cataloging in Publication Data
A catalog record for this book has been requested

ISBN 0–415–09971–4 (hbk)
ISBN 0–415–09972–2 (pbk)

Contents

Illustrations

FIGURES

TABLES

Contributors

Jonathan Bradshaw has been Professor of Social Policy and Head of the Department of Social Policy and Social Work at the University of York since 1988. He was founder and Director of the Social Policy Research Unit between 1973 and 1988. His main research interests are in family policy, energy and social policy, means-tested benefits, poverty, inequality and living standards, and he has published widely in these fields. He has been a member of the Child Poverty Action Group national executive, a member of the Social Security Research Policy Committee and an adviser to the Social Security Committee of the House of Commons. He is Director of the Department of Social Security Summer School, Chair of the Management Committee of North Yorkshire Welfare Benefits Unit, and a member of the Joseph Rowntree Foundation Social Policy Committee.

Carol Bryce is currently working in development and evaluation for the Health Education Board for Scotland. She was previously a Research Fellow in the Public Health Research Unit, University of Glasgow, where the children's accidents project was based. She is a geographer whose main interests are inequality and health. She has published on a variety of topics, including teacher recruitment, geographical health differences and children's accidents. Her current work focuses on nutrition, through which she has developed an interest in the sociology of food and eating.

Ray Fitzpatrick is a Fellow of Nuffield College, Oxford, and University Lecturer in Medical Sociology, University of Oxford. He is a co-editor of *The Experience of Illness* (Routledge, 1984) and co-edited with Anthony Hopkins *Measurement of Patients' Satisfaction with their Care* (Royal College of Physicians, 1993). He has been involved in a major longitudinal study of HIV prevalence and sexual behaviour in gay men.

Current research interests focus on patients' contributions to the evaluation of health care via measures of patient satisfaction, health status and quality of life. He is also co-editor with Stan Newman of a series of monographs published by Routledge – 'The Experience of Illness'.

Gerry Humphris is Lecturer at the Department of Clinical Psychology, University of Liverpool. He has carried out research in a variety of areas, including mental health promotion and health-needs assessment and is currently involved in a research project focusing on the experience of stress in junior doctors which is funded through the national Research and Development strategy.

David Hunter has been Director of the Nuffield Institute for Health, University of Leeds since 1989, and Professor of Health Policy and Management since July 1991. He is a non-executive director of Leeds Health Care Authority and has been an adviser to the House of Commons Social Services Committee on an inquiry into community care. From 1987 to 1988 he was a health policy analyst with the King's Fund Institute in London, and between 1982 and 1987 he led a five-year government funded research study on services for elderly people, based in the University of Aberdeen's Department of Community Medicine. He has published widely on aspects of health and social care policy and management practices, including the issue of rationing in health care. He is author of *Rationing Dilemmas in Healthcare*, a NAHAT research paper, and co-author of a forthcoming report on the same theme to be published by the Institute for Public Policy Research. He is co-author of *The Dynamics of British Health Policy* (Unwin Hyman, 1990), and of *Just Managing: Power and Culture in the NHS* (Macmillan, 1992). He contributes a monthly column to the *Health Service Journal*.

Andrew Long is Senior Lecturer in Health Systems Research at the Nuffield Institute for Health, University of Leeds, and Project Director of the UK Clearing House on Health Outcomes. He has taught and researched extensively in the areas of effectiveness, outcomes and evaluation in general.

Suzanne Moffatt is a Research Associate in the Department of Epidemiology and Public Health at the University of Newcastle upon Tyne, working on the relationship between industrial pollution and the health of nearby populations. Previously, she trained and worked as a Speech Therapist before doing a Ph.D. in Sociolinguistics at Newcastle University.

Bie Nio Ong is Senior Lecturer at the Centre for Health Planning and Management, Keele University. Her main research interests are modelling health needs assessment, outcome measurement and comparative health care. She is Director of the MBA (Health Executive) and the Diploma in Management (for women doctors) at the Centre and a non-executive director of an acute hospitals trust. She is author of *The Practice of Health Services Research* (Chapman & Hall, 1993).

Peter Phillimore lectures in Social Anthropology at the University of Newcastle upon Tyne. He has a Ph.D. from Durham University based on fieldwork in North India. In recent years he has been doing research on health and inequality, and health and industrial pollution, in north-east England and has published widely in these fields.

Jennie Popay is Professor of Community Health at the University of Salford and Director of the Public Health Research and Resource Centre (PHRRC), which was established by the NHS in 1991, with funding from Bolton, Salford, Trafford and Wigan Health Authorities and the NW Regional Health Authority. PHRRC has an extensive programme of health services research including various projects assessing health and social care needs from lay and clinical perspectives and measuring patients' assessment of the outcomes of care. Previously Senior Research Officer at the Thomas Coram Research Unit and before that a lecturer on the team for the Open University Course, Health and Disease, she has published widely in the health field. Her particular research interests include gender and social class inequalities in health, and the nature of relationships between lay and professional knowledge of health, illness and health care. Her recent publications include the edited collection (with Basiro Davey) *Dilemmas in Health Care* (Open University Press, 1993).

Cathie Rice has lived in Corkerhill for the last six years. Married to Joe, she has three children and was an active member of Corkerhill Community Council for four years, three of those as chair of the group. Now employed by the Safe Levern Pollock Project, a project aimed at addressing local safety issues, Cathie is less able to be involved fully but retains a lively interest in the local community.

Helen Roberts is head of research and development for Barnardo's, the largest voluntary child-care organization in the UK. With her co-authors she carried out the Corkerhill study, described in their chapter in this book, while employed as Senior Research Fellow in the Faculty of Medicine at the University of Glasgow. Her recent publications include the edited collections *Women's Health Counts* (Routledge, 1990) and *Women's*

Health Matters (Routledge, 1991). The book of the Corkerhill study, *Children at Risk?*, will be published by the Open University Press in 1994.

Gilbert Smith is Professor in the Department of Social Policy at the University of Hull, and has also been chair of a purchasing health authority. He has published widely in academic and policy journals.

Susan Smith is Professor of Geography at the University of Edinburgh. She has written widely on aspects of health, safety and social welfare. Her recent books include *Housing and Social Policy* (Macmillan, 1990) (co-authors David Clapham and Peter Kemp), *Housing for Health* (Longman, 1991) (co-editor) and *The Politics of Race and Residence* (Polity, 1989). Her current research includes a study of child accidents and a national survey of housing provision for people with health and mobility needs.

Meg Stacey, Emeritus Professor of Sociology at Warwick University, began her academic life as an Oxford University extra-mural tutor working with the Workers' Educational Association. As the result of this she published *Tradition and Change: A Study of Banbury* (Oxford University Press, 1960). She has focused on issues in the sociology of health for the past thirty years, editing *Hospitals, Children and their Families* (Routledge & Kegan Paul, 1970) and (with David Hall) *Beyond Separation: Further Studies of Children in Hospital* (Routledge & Kegan Paul, 1979), and writing *The Sociology of Health and Healing* (Unwin Hyman, 1988). She served on the Welsh Hospital Board, the Michael Davies Committee on Hospital Complaints Procedure and, as a lay member, on the General Medical Council. From this derives *Regulating British Medicine: The General Medical Council* (Wiley, 1992). She continues to be an engaged sociologist.

Gareth Williams is Reader in the Sociology of Health and Illness in the Department of Sociology, University of Salford. He has carried out research on the experiences of chronic illness and has a particular interest in the nature of lay knowledge and the politics of public participation. He has published extensively in medical and sociological journals. He is currently involved in projects looking at different aspects of health service reforms and their effects on the delivery of health care. He is co-editor (with Steven Platt, Sue Scott and Hilary Thomas) of *Private Risks and Public Dangers* (Avebury, 1992) and *Locating Health* (Avebury, 1993); and (with Jon Gabe and David Kelleher) of *Challenging Medicine* (Routledge, 1994).

Preface

Health and health care are no longer the preserves of specialists. Those whose occupation it is to provide health care, to research the causes and consequences of health and illness or to frame health policies, are increasingly being called upon to justify what they do or fail to do, and what they say or do not say, within a much larger arena. A Secretary of State for Health can expect to be on television and radio with greater frequency than her or his counterpart in the Foreign Office. Professors of health services management write guest columns for the *British Medical Journal* and the *Guardian* newspaper with equal ease. And the media airwaves are filled with *vox pop* soundbites from experts – professional and lay – on every conceivable aspect of human ill-health and the organization of health care. When even literary periodicals provide space for comment on health care we can be sure that health is well and truly a public issue (Pimlott 1993).

For those whose job it is to make sense of what goes on in the world of health, there are now many more actors on the set whom the observer needs to watch and listen to. Researching the people's health means attending to many voices and making use of multiple perspectives. This volume attempts to provide some understanding of what this involves.

The chapters in this book were all originally papers delivered to a series of seminars, held in 1992 and 1993, funded by the King's Fund and by the Economic and Social Research Council (ESRC award number A451 26 400224) and collectively entitled *Social Research in Public Health*. The objectives of the seminar series were twofold:

1 to address some of the key methodological, theoretical, and policy issues in the field of public health research, and
2 to provide a bridge between the academic and the health-service worlds – between the doers and the users of research.

There were times when the voices at these seminars were so numerous, the languages so various, and professional interests so cherished, that building bridges seemed a hopeless project. But there were other occasions on which views coalesced and arguments were carried forward in a way that opened up exciting possibilities for research, policy and practice. As the seminar series progressed it became clear to us that a key area of concern was the importance of lay knowledge about health and illness, and the relationships between lay people, social scientists and other orthodox experts in the context of changing ideas about public health and the organization of health services. It is to that area of concern that this volume is devoted.

We believe this to be a timely book. In the context of the challenges orthodox medicine currently faces (Gabe *et al.* 1994), and the political investment that has now been built up in a health service driven by the needs of users rather than the interests of professionals, the emphasis on the ways in which we can develop research within health services that draws on the perspectives of the many interested parties that make up 'the people' is of very great importance. It is hoped that the book will appeal not only to sociologists and other social scientists, but also to those working in health services, and those people, often called 'consumers', who are also experts on the origins of ill-health and the principal producers of health care.

We are grateful to Chris Saunders, Angela Greenall, Ursula Harries and Sue Smart for help in organizing the seminars and preparing this book for press; and to Andrew Long and David Hunter of the Nuffield Institute for Health at Leeds, for hosting the seminar on 'Outcomes for Health'.

Jennie Popay and Gareth Williams

REFERENCES

Gabe, J., Kelleher, D., and Williams, G., eds (1994) *Challenging Medicine*, London: Routledge.

Pimlott, B. (1993) 'Towards the welfare state: Clinton's health plan and the new social democracy', *Times Literary Supplement* 19 November 4729: 15–16.

Introduction

Jennie Popay and Gareth Williams

> Real change in the modern age requires not the seizure of power, the revolutionary's dream, but the dispersal of power . . . it must be inspired by a sense of the common good or democracy becomes 'boring fragile and weak'.
>
> (Lewis 1990)

CHANGING IDEAS ABOUT HEALTH AND ILLNESS

Towards the close of the twentieth century, researching the people's health seems an ever more complex and uncertain endeavour. Nonetheless, despite the uncertainties with which we are faced, two developments seem to be taking shape. One is the growing importance of the role of social scientists, and the other is the need to take seriously people's own views about their health and their health needs. This book is about these developments, and each chapter provides a different illustration of their significance, and the factors that may liberate or inhibit them.

At the end of the last century, research into the health of the people was primarily concerned with the physical environment of climate and soil and, increasingly, the socially constructed natural environment of buildings, dwellings and habitations (Armstrong 1993). Public health, or sanitary science, was directed towards understanding and controlling the mechanisms of transmission of substances between bodies and environments, particularly as they related to the spread of infectious diseases, and working out ways in which basic levels of health could be protected and enhanced through various forms of social engineering (Webster 1990).

One hundred years later the world is dramatically divided – contemporary public health is a tale of two regions. In the 'underdeveloped' parts of the world, the picture looks remarkably similar to that of the last century, even where the causes of their health problems are the result of profoundly different and transglobal processes (Gray 1993). In Western industrialized areas, by contrast, there has been a metamorphosis in patterns of health and illness.

Although the labelling of diseases as 'new' and 'old' is rather simplistic (*Lancet* 1993), unprecedented improvements in living conditions such as diet, housing, and sanitation, along with demographic changes producing the ageing of populations, have had a profound impact on the health profile of Western societies. Chronic illnesses have replaced infectious diseases as the major cause of mortality and morbidity, and their social sequelae – disability and handicap (World Health Organization 1980) or quality of life – are of prime importance in any assessment of 'the people's health' in the Western world.

These changes in patterns of health and illness have led to the need for aetiological models which encompass the social and psychological as well as the physical environment, and which incorporate factors relating to culture and lifestyle. During the 1970s and 1980s, the idea that individuals are responsible for their own health became the prominent motif of health policy (Department of Health and Social Security 1977). The idea that individuals could, through their own actions, do something to avoid heart attacks, and that families could, through careful dietary management, engender significant improvements in health rapidly became part of a new orthodoxy (Allsop 1984). To some extent this new orthodoxy can be seen as the anxious response of governments to the fiscal crisis of the State (O'Connor 1973), to which the costs of health care were making a significant input. However, among commentators across the political spectrum, there was also a growing disillusionment with the record and the prospects of curative medicine (Allsop 1984); and a culture of anti-professionalism within which doctors were characterized as more controlling than caring (Zola 1972; Illich 1977; Kennedy 1981).

Within public health, a 'new public health' emerged, influenced initially by the Lalonde Report in Canada (Lalonde 1974) and later by the World Health Organization's *Targets for Health for All* (1985). These statements emphasized 'refocusing upstream', intersectoral collaboration, and community participation in public health initiatives (Ashton and Seymour 1988). In the context of these ideological developments, the centres of orthodox public health surveillance began to switch their focus towards 'lifestyle' and the social environment (Etheridge 1992). Over the same period, the relationships between lifestyle, the environment and health were given a new twist by the arrival of 'new' communicable diseases, notably AIDS. These have stirred profound anxieties about infection and contagion that hark back to earlier periods (Frankenberg 1988; Ranger and Slack 1992).

And it is not just AIDS. Outbreaks of legionnaire's disease and salmonella poisoning gave rise to the Acheson inquiry into communicable disease and the public health function (Secretary of State for Social Services 1987), and led some commentators to perceive the 're-invention of public health' (*Lancet* 1988). A series of 'scares' regarding food-borne infections have taken place in recent years, and these have undermined confidence in the viability of the food chain, which is normally taken for granted.

Moreover, diseases which had been regarded as dead long ago in Western societies, such as tuberculosis (Watson 1993) and rickets, are once more raising their heads. The effects of the globalization of economic systems, therefore, can be seen in both the huge disparities in health and wealth between 'north' and 'south', and in the widening health gap between different social strata within British society (Smith and Egger 1993).

QUESTIONING HEALTH CARE SYSTEMS

Alongside the changing pattern of ill-health, medical care has become increasingly sophisticated and highly technical. Paralleling this there is growing concern at the cost and appropriateness of the existing balance between primary and secondary services – between prevention, care and treatment. More generally, there is widespread questioning of the paternalist philosophies and statist welfare structures and philosophies established at the end of the Second World War. Countries as diverse as Britain, Holland, Sweden and New Zealand are pursuing similar goals in the health and welfare field with the introduction of markets and a shift in emphasis towards primary care (Ham and Calltrop 1992). These and many other countries are developing similar strategies to rein in expenditure (Flynn 1992). In the lexicon of public health, prioritization and preference are to be found where sanitation and control were a century ago.

Against this background there are various ways in which the power, status and knowledge of the medical profession, for so long virtually taken for granted, are being challenged from both inside and outside the health care system (Gabe *et al.* 1994). In Britain, but also elsewhere (Ashton 1993; Caplan 1993), this is the decade of the consumer and 'managed competition' in health care. In country after country, the rhetoric of health care reforms emphasizes the importance of developing services which are based on knowledge about health and social-care needs, rather than the interests of different health professionals. In reality, of course, this emphasis on needs-based services has to be seen in the context of finite resources and the calls for targeting and prioritization, and is subservient to them.

CONTINUITY AND CHANGE

Alongside all this change some things have remained remarkably constant. Economic inequalities are persistent in industrialized societies. As an editorial in the *British Medical Journal* put it: 'The classless society anticipated by Mr Major has had an extended gestation, which shows no sign of ending' (Smith and Egger 1993: 1085).

The distribution of income and wealth has changed little over the past fifty years in most richer countries and in some instances has grown more unequal (Plotnick 1993; Pond and Popay 1993; Wilkinson 1989). Japan is a notable exception, becoming over the years more equal. In contemporary Britain, around a quarter of the population is living on incomes at or below the 'poverty line' (Oppenheim 1993).

Social inequalities in the experience of ill-health in Western societies mimic socio-economic differentials in Britain and other Western societies (Wilkinson 1992; Dahl and Kjaersgaard 1993; Wennemo 1993). While these inequalities in the most basic of life chances – expected longevity at birth – may vary in scale, they persist across industrial societies. People born into higher social classes (however measured) have a lower mortality rate at all ages and for all causes than those born into lower social classes (Townsend and Davidson 1982). In recent years other dimensions of health inequalities – related, for example, to gender, ethnicity, age and geographical area, and to morbidity as well as mortality – have also been highlighted in research (Popay *et al.* 1993; Smith *et al.* 1990; Whitehead 1987; Townsend *et al.* 1988; Eames *et al.* 1993; Andrews and Jewson 1993). There may be room for debate about the extent to which post-Second World War welfare provision in Western societies has ameliorated these inequalities, but there is no doubt that it has failed to remove them. There is also evidence that these inequalities too may have increased in recent years (Smith and Egger 1993; Phillimore *et al.* 1994). It is to be expected that this social polarization forms an important context for the return of diseases of poverty, such as rickets and tuberculosis, to 'richer' countries.

A final intriguing element of contemporary health concerns is the re-emergence of the environment as a source of risk across the 'developed' world (Doll 1992; *Lancet* 1992). Indeed, so endemic are these risks perceived to be that sociologists have begun to identify the emergence of a 'risk society' (Beck 1992). While aetiological explanations for contemporary disease patterns in industrial societies tend to focus on lifestyles and psycho-social factors, the health hazards of the physical environment, mediated through economic policies, are once again increasing in prominence (Porter and Porter 1990). There are increasing instances of public concern over environmental toxins (see Phillimore and Moffatt in this volume; Brown and Mikkelsen 1990; Williams and Popay 1994). These also highlight public suspicion of the professional experts entrusted with protecting the people's health. At the same time, however, some medical experts have helped raise the alarm against powerful non-medical interests, whether car manufacturers, polluting industries, public housing design, etc. The new public health movement emphasizes the need for community participation and development alongside traditional professional interventions to promote health (Ashton and Seymour 1988), and numerous local examples of intersectoral and participative working now exist.

CHANGING APPROACHES TO RESEARCHING THE PEOPLE'S HEALTH

In some respects, therefore, the people's health, the services developed to protect and enhance it, and the status of the professionals to whom this responsibility was entrusted are in a state of flux. Around the globe, policy changes are under way on a scale and of a nature unprecedented since the wave of reforms in the 1940s. At the same time, however, it is apparent that health and social inequalities persist. In the face of this imbroglio, serious doubts have been cast on the relevance of traditional approaches to researching the people's health. These doubts are woven out of a number of strands.

First, many of the analytical problems raised by chronic disease, AIDS, food-borne infections and environmental pollutants are forcing researchers to accept the limitations of existing models of aetiology and to consider other ways of exploring the relationship between the social and the physical environment, individual behaviour and ill-health. In the context of social inequalities in mortality, for instance, it has recently been argued that: 'attempting to explain inequalities in any simple sense may be futile, while the concept of "cause" used in its usual epidemiological sense is probably inadequate' (Smith and Egger 1993:

1086). Although, to some extent, these arguments echo a similar public health critique mounted in the 1920s and 1930s, new theoretical, conceptual and methodological tools and perspectives can now be brought to bear on contemporary problems in researching the people's health (Long 1993). Above all, interdisciplinary collaboration is required if causal relationships are to be adequately mapped and understood.

Second, the significance of lay knowledge about health, illness and care is increasingly recognized. Such knowledge has to be a vital component of our understanding of the experience of ill-health and of the processes and outcomes of health and social care. However, traditional, epidemiological research methods are unable to provide us with avenues to make this knowledge accessible, and the consequences of the failure to integrate local, informal knowledge into scientific evaluation and decision-making can be serious (Wynne 1991). Research methods are needed which will allow 'lay' experts to be involved in the design and conduct of research and which will allow their voices to be heard directly. As one social scientist argues: 'Public health researchers must begin to devise methodologies and theories which allow for genuine participation in the research process' (Kelly 1990: 9).

Third, health care systems are rightly the target for much research effort concerned with the people's health, yet the average health service researcher is ill-equipped for the job. Whilst the evaluation of interventions should remain of prime importance, it has already been argued that the evaluation must shift to involve lay perspectives. More importantly, evaluative research is only one dimension of the research agenda facing contemporary health care systems, and this broader agenda demands a portfolio of theories and methods. There is an urgent need to re-tool health service researchers and to encourage greater tolerance of difference and diversity amongst those involved (Pope and Mays 1993).

THE CONTOURS OF THE BOOK

These then are the themes that run through the contributions in this book. There are four parts, and the first begins with two chapters exploring the health service context for research on the people's health.

In the first chapter, David Hunter maps out the prospects for social research in the aftermath of the National Health Service (NHS) reforms of the 1990s. He suggests that in addition to the impact of the reforms themselves, social science has an important contribution to make to research into health needs assessment, the measurement of effectiveness, and outcomes and user involvement. However, he argues that it is not self-evident that social scientists have the ability to respond to the challenge of contemporary changes in health and social-care policy and practice. If they are to do so, then difficult issues within and between social-science disciplines will have to be resolved.

In the following chapter, Gilbert Smith, Jennie Popay and Gareth Williams focus more sharply on research into health needs and health care outcomes. They ask what it will require from social scientists and managers alike if research-based knowledge is to drive health care systems. Drawing on Smith's experience as chair of a purchasing health authority, they consider how this process will be influenced by the 'quasi-market' forces now developing in the NHS. Though the issues in these two chapters are viewed through the lens of the British NHS, they are relevant to those involved in health services research in other countries.

The concept and measurement of health needs are the subject of the second part of the book. Here Jonathan Bradshaw revisits his celebrated and widely used typology of need (Bradshaw 1972), and critically assesses the relevance of the concept for contemporary public health research. Briefly reviewing different perspectives on need – the philosopher's, the economist's and the politician's – he concludes that whilst the 1990s appear to be the 'decade of need' this amounts, in the political sphere at least, to a 'cynical adulteration of the concept'. For 'need' in the 1990s, he suggests, one should read targeting, while what is required is a renewed emphasis within research on the utility of the concept of inequality.

Notwithstanding the considerable theoretical, methodological and political difficulties, Bie Nio Ong and Gerry Humphris argue in their chapter that research focusing on health 'needs' can be policy-relevant but that much thought must go into the method to be used. They suggest that Rapid Appraisal (RA) methodologies, which are increasingly being used within the NHS, provide an appropriate approach. These methods, they argue, allow both the purchasers and the providers of health care to listen to what local people have to say, and to involve them in the joint definition of need, priority-setting and evaluation.

The third part of the book spotlights lay knowledge about health and illness and considers its nature and significance along a number of dimensions. In her contribution on the power of lay knowledge, Meg Stacey provides an account, simultaneously autobiographical and sociological, of the triumphs and frustrations experienced by lay people involved in fighting to protect or enhance the services they need. The many struggles by local people in Britain in the 1980s to prevent the closure of accident and emergency departments, or to oppose the development of hospital trusts, represent lay knowledge in action. Many of the examples Stacey uses come from the women's movement. She examines these in relation to what she sees as two key assumptions: that all people are of equal worth, and that people are producers as well as consumers of health care. On this basis she draws our attention to three key themes: the nature of the knowledge upon which ordinary people and professionals draw, the relationships between different kinds of knowledge, and the workings of power and knowledge in people–professional relationships.

Stacey is primarily concerned with the power of lay knowledge in health services. In our contribution we broaden the focus to consider issues on the public health research agenda. We explore the limitations of traditional epidemiology as a tool for understanding the genesis of contemporary health problems and in identifying the health needs of local populations. Using an example from environmental health of a local community taking action against the pollution of their water supply, we illustrate the depth of disagreement that can emerge between professionals and local people. We go on to argue that sociological research, because of its methodological and theoretical pluralism, has a major role to play in the new health care arena. Whatever the economic and political forces underlying the rediscovery of the voice of the local citizen, one of its cultural effects has been to create the expectation that health authorities and other agencies should listen and respond to a multitude of local voices and opinions.

The next two chapters provide fuller examinations of the problems lay people can have when they try to get their understanding and knowledge of health problems taken seriously. These chapters also provide different models for the involvement of social scientists in researching the people's health.

In their chapter Cathie Rice and her colleagues discuss the potentially fruitful collaboration that can take place between social scientists and a local community – in this case, in relation to the problem of child safety in dangerous urban environments. The chapter describes some of the social context and relationships contained in a study of child accidents and the maintenance of safety which ran alongside a parents' action group on child safety in Corkerhill, a housing estate in Glasgow. The study shows how communities are well placed to recognize the dangers surrounding them, and how this knowledge should be used to make the environment safer.

Peter Phillimore and Suzanne Moffatt focus on another type of danger that urban, industrial societies contain. Their chapter is about the role of the knowledge and beliefs of local people in guiding epidemiological studies of the relationship between air pollution from industrial sites and the health of people living nearby. Using two case studies conducted in the industrial north-east of England, one on Tyneside and the other on Teesside, they explore the relationships between local people, researchers and various other agencies and organizations involved. They argue that it is all too easy to discount the voices of local people in such studies, on supposedly 'sound' methodological grounds. However, like Rice and her colleagues, Phillimore and Moffatt insist that the knowledge of local communities is *expert* knowledge in the sense that it is based on direct day-to-day experience and that the voices of the people must make themselves heard in both research and policy.

The fourth and final part of the book returns to one of the central concerns of contemporary health care systems: how to conceptualize and measure the health and social outcomes of the treatments and interventions that patients receive. How do we know when a health service input has done any good? In chronic illness, for example, the goal may be to improve the functioning of the patient or to increase ability to cope with pain and handicap, rather than cure her or his disease.

In his useful overview Andrew Long considers the issues that have made the assessment of outcomes an urgent policy concern in the UK – the drive to cost containment, for example, and the development of a national health strategy. He goes on to look at the problems involved in defining and measuring outcome, and in developing a workable method of assessing health and social outcome in routine clinical settings. Long notes that the problems will only be overcome when professionals move beyond their own disciplinary perspectives and work collaboratively with other scientists as well as users and consumers of health care.

Ray Fitzpatrick notes the extent of the challenge that chronic illness poses to the logic of epidemiological methods. In essence, the incidence and prevalence of disease do not map in any simple way on to the need for health care. For this reason, he argues, the social sciences have an enormous contribution to make to assessing health need and the outcomes of care. In particular, he notes the distinctive contributions social science has already made to our understanding of chronic illness, contributions which have emphasized the importance of looking at the illness from the ill person's own perspective. Fitzpatrick reviews various approaches to the assessment of health need and health status in chronic illness; examines their sensitivity to the subtleties and peculiarities of chronic illnesses; and considers the extent to which they can be used in population and clinical contexts in a way that does justice to the perspectives and concerns of patients.

CONCLUDING COMMENT

All the contributions to this book have at their heart two key questions. What contribution can social science make to the rapidly changing world of health and health services? And how can this contribution work to ensure that lay perspectives are accorded (in Stacey's terms) 'equal worth'? The danger is that social scientists either take all views as 'equal', in a naive calculus, and fail to recognize the continuing need for some kind of resolution of differences in open and democratic public debate (Habermas 1989; Beck 1992). Or, having genuflected to the 'value' of lay views, they retreat, along with their colleagues in public health and epidemiology, into some 'final analysis' in which 'science' is the bedrock.

Those who spend their time pondering the contours of 'high modernity' (Giddens 1991) may smile, shrug their shoulders, and murmur 'c'est la vie post-moderne'. Those who spend their working lives at the intersections of theory, research, policy and practice have no such escape. And amongst those for whom the closure of a ward, an accident and emergency department, or a whole hospital means something more than the deconstruction of a discursive practice, these questions will have continuing and urgent relevance.

REFERENCES

Allsop, J. (1984) *Health Policy and the National Health Service*, London: Longman.

Andrews, A., and Jewson, N. (1993) 'Ethnicity and infant deaths: the implications of recent statistical evidence for materialist explanations', *Sociology of Health and Illness* 15: 137–56.

Armstrong, D. (1993) 'Public health spaces and the fabrication of identity', *Sociology* 27: 393–410.

Ashton, J., and Seymour, H. (1988) *The New Public Health*, Milton Keynes: Open University Press.

Ashton, T. (1993) 'From evolution to revolution: restructuring the New Zealand health system', *Health Care Analysis* 1: 57–62.

Beck, U. (1992) *Risk Society: Towards a New Modernity*, London: Sage.

Bradshaw, J. (1972) 'A taxonomy of social need', in McLachlan, G. (ed.) *Problems and Progress in Medical Care*, Oxford: Nuffield Provincial Hospitals Trust.

Brown, P., and Mikkelsen, E.J. (1990) *No Safe Place: Toxic Waste, Leukemia, and Community Action*, Berkeley: University of California Press.

Caplan, A. (1993) 'Clinton's health care reforms', *British Medical Journal* 307: 813–14.

Dahl, E., and Kjaersgaard, P. (1993) 'Trends in socioeconomic mortality differentials in post-war Norway: evidence and interpretations', *Sociology of Health and Illness* 15: 587–611.

Department of Health and Social Security (1977) *Prevention and Health: Everybody's Business*, London: HMSO.

Doll, R. (1992) 'Health and the environment in the 1990s', *American Journal of Public Health*, 82: 933–43.

Eames, M., Ben-Shiomo, Y., and Marmot, M.G. (1993) 'Social deprivation and preventive mortality: regional comparison across England', *British Medical Journal*, 307: 1097–102.

Etheridge, E.W. (1992) *Sentinel for Health: A History of the Centers for Disease Control*, Berkeley and Los Angeles: University of California Press.

Flynn, R. (1992) *Structures of Power and Control in Health Management*, London, Routledge.

Frankenberg, R. (1988) 'AIDS and the anthropologists', *Anthropology Today* 4: 13–15.

Gabe, J., Kelleher, D., and Williams G., eds (1994) *Challenging Medicine*, London: Routledge.

Giddens, A. (1991) *The Consequences of Modernity*, Cambridge: Polity Press.

Gray, A. (1993) *World Health and Disease*, Milton Keynes: Open University Press in association with the Open University.

Habermas, J. (1989) *The Structural Transformation of the Public Sphere: An Inquiry into a Category of Bourgeois Society*, Cambridge: Polity Press.

Ham, C., and Calltrop, J. (1992) 'Money Money Money', *Health Service Journal* 102, 5295: 22–5.

Illich, I. (1977) *The Limits to Medicine*, Harmondsworth: Penguin Books.

Kelly, M.P. (1990) 'The role of research in the new public health', *Critical Public Health* 3: 4–9.

Kennedy, I. (1981) *Unmasking Medicine*, London: Allen & Unwin.

Lalonde, M. (1974) *A New Perspective on the Health of Canadians*, Ottawa: Ministry of Supply and Services.

Lancet (1988) 'Back to the future – the reinvention of public health', *The Lancet* 339: 1157–9.

—— (1992) 'Environmental pollution: it kills trees but does it kill people?', *The Lancet* 340: 821–2.

—— (1993) 'Rise and fall of diseases', *The Lancet* 341: 151–2.

Lewis, F. (1990) 'Needs of civil society' (editorial), *The New York Times*, 8 August.

Long, A. (1993) *Understanding Health and Disease: Towards a Knowledge Base for Public Health Action*, Report of a workshop, 30 June – 2 July 1993, Leeds: Nuffield Institute for Health.

O'Connor, J. (1973) *The Fiscal Crisis of the State*, London: St Martin's Press.

Oppenheim, C. (1993) *Poverty: The Facts*, London: Child Poverty Action Group.

Phillimore, P., Beattie, A., and Townsend, P. (1994) 'Widening inequality of health in northern England 1981–91', *British Medical Journal* 308: 1125–8.

Plotnick, R.D. (1993) 'Changes in poverty, income inequality and the standard of living in the United States during the Reagan years', *International Journal of Health Services,* 23: 347–58.

Pond, C., and Popay, J. (1993) 'Poverty, economic inequality and health', in Davey, B., and Popay, J., eds, *Dilemmas in Health Care*, Birmingham: Open University Press.

Popay, J., Bartley, M., and Owen, C. (1993) 'Gender inequalities in health: social position, affective disorders and minor morbidity', *Social Science and Medicine* 36: 21–32.

Pope, C., and Mays, N. (1993) 'Opening the black box: an encounter in the corridors of health services research', *British Medical Journal* 306: 315–18

Porter, D., and Porter, R. (1990) 'The ghost of Edwin Chadwick', *British Medical Journal* 301: 252.

Ranger T., and Slack P., eds (1992) *Epidemics and Ideas: Essays on the Historical Perception of Pestilence*, Cambridge: Cambridge University Press.

Secretary of State for Social Services (1987) *Public Health in England: the Report of the Committee of Inquiry into the Development of the Public Health Function* (Chair: Sir D. Acheson), London: HMSO.

Smith, G. Davey, Bartley, M., and Blane, D. (1990) 'The Black Report on socio-economic inequalities in health 10 years on', *British Medical Journal* 301: 373–7.

Smith, G. Davey, and Egger, M. (1993) 'Socio-economic differentials in wealth and health', *British Medical Journal* 307: 1085–86.

Townsend, P., and Davidson, N. (1982) *Inequalities in Health: The Black Report*, Harmondsworth: Penguin Books.

Townsend, P., Phillimore, P., and Beattie, A. (1988) *Health and Deprivation: Inequalities and the North*, London: Croom Helm.

Watson J.M. (1993) 'Tuberculosis in Britain today' (editorial), *British Medical Journal* 306: 221–2.

Webster C. (1990) *The Victorian Public Health Legacy: A Challenge to the Future*, Birmingham: The Public Health Alliance.

Wennemo, I. (1993) 'Infant mortality, public policy, and inequality: a comparison of 18 industrialised countries', *Sociology of Health and Illness* 15: 429–46.

Whitehead, M. (1987) *The Health Divide: Inequalities in Health in the 1980s*, London, Health Education Council.

Wilkinson, R.G. (1989) 'Class mortality differentials, income distribution and trends in poverty 1921–1981, *Journal of Social Policy* 18: 307–35.

—— (1992) 'Income distribution and life expectancy', *British Medical Journal* 304: 165–68.

Williams, G., and Popay, J. (1994) 'Lay knowledge and the privilege of experience', in Gabe, J., Kelleher, D., and Williams, G., eds, *Challenging Medicine*, London: Routledge.

World Health Organization (1980) *International Classification of Impairments, Disabilities, and Handicaps*, Geneva: World Health Organization.

—— (1985) *Targets for Health for All*, Copenhagen: World Health Organization.

Wynne, B. (1991) 'After Chernobyl: science made too simple?' *New Scientist*, 26 January: 44–6.

Zola, I.K. (1972) 'Medicine as an institution of social control: the medicalizing of society', *The Sociological Review* 20: 487–504.

Part I

Social research and the National Health Service reforms in the 1990s

Chapter 1

Social research and health policy in the aftermath of the NHS reforms

David Hunter

INTRODUCTION

In 1991 unprecedented reforms were introduced into the British National Health Service (NHS) and the related sectors of primary health and community care. Whatever the merits and demerits of these reforms, they represent both a major challenge and an opportunity to the social research community. There are issues about what precisely the challenge amounts to, whether social scientists are in a position to meet the challenge, and what needs to happen to maximize the undoubted opportunities which exist. These issues ultimately go beyond the confines of the social research community since it is in the interests of better public policy that research be commissioned and that its fruits inform the policy-making process.

This chapter is in three sections, each dealing with the principal themes just noted: the nature of the challenge facing social research; the ability of social scientists to meet the challenge, and how social scientists can seize the initiative.

THE CHALLENGE

The challenge presented to social science research by the health and social care reforms has two elements: first, the nature of the reform process itself and the changes it has triggered; and, second, the desired outcomes which the changes are ostensibly directed towards securing. The rest of this section examines each element in turn.

The reform process

As Kenneth Clarke, a former Secretary of State for Health, put it when announcing the NHS reforms in the House of Commons at the end of January 1989, the changes amount to the most formidable programme of reform since the inception of the Service (Secretaries of State for Health, Wales, Northern Ireland and Scotland 1989). Unlike earlier reforms in the NHS's history, the changes on this occasion are different in kind. They are not fundamentally about 'boxes and charts', nor are they concerned with merely rearranging the organizational furniture. They are directed at the very processes involved in 'doing the business' within the NHS and related sectors. To this end, the changes are expressly aimed at disturbing the chemistry of the NHS and, in particular, at challenging some of the professional, managerial and organizational routines and standard operating procedures which have persisted over the years.

The intention is to shift the power relations between the principal actors, notably doctors and managers. The motivation for such a strategy lay in a complex of frustrations, which came to a head in late 1987. These included: repeated clamouring from vested interests, principally the medical profession, for more resources – the 'chorus of complaint' Enoch Powell wrote of (Powell 1966); political dogma concerning the very existence of public sector monopolies; a zealous faith in the virtues of the market-place; and a penchant for seeking managerial quick fixes to intractable problems over resource allocation and priority-setting. This latter strategy owes more to image management than anything more substantive or lasting by way of change.

This is not the place to rehearse the NHS reforms, or those in primary and social care, in any detail. (For a review, see Harrison, *et al.* 1990; Harrison, *et al.* 1992; Davey and Popay 1993.) The term 'NHS reforms' is used loosely to embrace the changes occurring not only in the NHS but also in primary care and community care. Never before in the history of these services have so much change and turbulence been unleashed simultaneously.

There are many aspects of the reforms which pose interesting research questions, and indeed some work, though probably not enough, is already in hand to address some of them. The potential items on a research agenda are listed in Figure 1.1. The list of issues, themes, questions and puzzles is almost limitless and can be rapidly assembled. What is interesting about any such list is the mix it is likely to contain of issues which have been around for years (e.g. coordinated service provision) and of new ones whose impact can only be guessed at (e.g. purchasing for health gain). The lexicon of health reform is substantially new. Whether it will have a substantive impact on the health care system remains to be seen.

- The purchaser–provider split in health and social care and its implications for planning and managing
- The aims of the purchasing role: purchasing for what? Health gain? Rationing?
- The incentives/disincentives introduced by general practitioner (GP) fundholding practices and their impact on referral behaviour, user preferences and access to care
- Needs assessment in local communities and among professionals
- The emergence of new interfaces between primary care, hospital care and community care and, possibly, a new set of perverse incentives as new forms of 'cost shunting' (i.e. shifting the responsibility from one agency on to another agency's budget) become attractive
- Moves towards new models of health agencies, e.g. purchasing consortia comprising district health authorities (DHAs) and family health services authorities (FHSAs), locality purchasing
- The meaning and realization of a mixed economy of care and its implications for traditional public sector organizations and management cultures and responsibilities
- The place of the consumer/user: empowered or exploited? Active or passive?
- The nature and operation of an internal market – or, more accurately, a provider market – and its relationship to a health strategy
- The changing frontier between medicine and management: does clinical autonomy mean anything any more – if it ever did?
- The role of health authorities as 'champions of the people': is this more than a slogan?
- The role of public health: is it about to undergo a renaissance or be absorbed by other specialists or groups?

Figure 1.1 The NHS reforms: a possible research agenda

Moreover, the language is evershifting to reflect the changing nuances of political discourse. There has been a metamorphosis since 1989 from the robust language of business, markets and contracts to the softer, more caring language of health gain, enabling and service agreements (Hunter 1993a). The harsher edge given to the reforms at their birth has been replaced by a more conciliatory, soothing terminology. A new vocabulary is being fashioned, and any analysis of the reforms will need to reflect this if the changes are to be fully captured and understood. A key area of concern is the increasingly blurred boundary between the public and private sectors. NHS trusts, for instance, occupy a 'twilight zone' between the public and private sectors. There is also the changing nature of public agencies as they withdraw from direct service provision and become enablers and regulators of service provided by others. What are the implications of these massive shifts for the way in which such agencies operate and conceive of their role?

Desired outcomes

The point to emphasize from the above account is the essentially *process*-orientated thrust of the reforms. They are primarily concerned with *means* rather than *ends.* They are intentionally aimed at reconfiguring relationships between users, providers and managers – or, to adopt Alford's (1975) over-used categories, the repressed interests, the professional monopolizers, and the corporate rationalizers – in ways which cannot be, and have not been, predicted.

The NHS 1989 White Paper barely mentioned public health (Secretaries of State for Health, Wales, Northern Ireland and Scotland 1989). The clear thrust of the NHS changes at the time of the White Paper was consumerist in the context of a market for services. But, more recently, as a result of the publication of the Health of the Nation strategy (Department of Health 1992a) and the strong emphasis on effective purchasing (Mawhinney and Nichol 1993), the reforms have been intent upon improving the health of the population by meeting its health needs, including hitherto unmet needs. The conceptual and organizational complexities involved in attempting to achieve these potentially conflicting policy ends defy contemplation, and it remains to be seen how committed to the purchasing role ministers prove to be.

DHAs confront a potentially unresolved tension: on the one hand they exist to meet demand for hospital services, and on the other they are expected to relate the distribution of their resources to their measurable (monitorable) impact on the health of the population (Harrison *et al.* 1989). This conflict between an individualistic ethos and a collectivist one could result in the neglect of an investment in health as pressures and potential perverse incentives in the system divert attention from a wider strategic view of health. The urgent may continue to drive out the important.

It was David Mellor, when Minister of Health, who said that the government did not know what the NHS would look like in five or ten years' time, but this, he claimed, would be a measure of the success of the reforms. The hallmark of the reform strategy is 'learning by doing'. As such it is evolving almost daily as rules of engagement between various groups are negotiated and become codified. The unfolding of the reforms in this way represents a major challenge to the social research community and places a premium on an awareness of the political and organizational context in which the reforms are being played out. Do researchers appreciate this? Can they rise to the challenge? Will anyone listen or care if they do or do not?

MEETING THE CHALLENGE

Successive reforms of the NHS, and moves to refocus health care priorities, from the early 1970s have helped spawn a modest body of research on the organizational, managerial and behaviourial aspects of the various changes. (For a brief review, see Hunter 1988; Harrison *et al.* 1992.) But this growth has been somewhat haphazard and uncoordinated. Moreover, it has not been matched by an increase in the ability of social research to inform or influence policy in any direct or explicit way. As Klein (1990: 501) has noted: 'successive governments . . . have seemingly undervalued, underfinanced, and underused the capacity of the research community to inform policy making'.

It is a view with which I have considerable sympathy. As I have argued elsewhere: 'social science research has failed to inform any of the changes in the organisation of the NHS over the past 14 years or so, and has also failed to establish the validity of the claims of reformers'. (Hunter 1988: 538).

Similarly, a former Permanent Secretary at the Department of Health (DoH), Sir Kenneth Stowe, reflecting on his time at the centre, concluded that the connection between health services research and the formulation of government policy is minimal (Stowe 1989: 502).

The place, and negligible contribution in the UK, of social research in general and health services research in particular, is a reflection of the low esteem in which research generally is held. While during the 1970s there was a perception that social research was being taken less seriously than it should, the 1980s witnessed a dramatic volte-face and the virtual dismissal of social research as being of no practical value. A partial exception was the (unfounded) legitimacy accorded inquiry by health economists into matters of health service costs, efficiency and value for money. What do the 1990s hold for social research? In a surprising break with the tradition of virtually ignoring the potential contribution of research, the community care White Paper devotes four paragraphs to the 'important contribution' of research 'to the effective design and delivery of community care services' (Secretaries of State for Health, Social Security, Wales and Scotland 1989, para. 5.31, 46). While such an endorsement of the value of research is to be applauded, the issue is rather more complicated.

Klein (1990) argues that social research in the UK has suffered from the existence of a monolithic and corporatist policy community which has remained largely impregnable to researchers or to the findings of research. He goes on to suggest that there is no obvious role for research in a setting where a widespread consensus exists among the various interests in the health policy community. He maintains that the situation is poised to change as critical scrutiny of the NHS, in particular clinical practices within it and the whole emphasis on health outcomes, gathers pace following the implementation of the NHS reforms. Of course, while such a 'breaking of the mould' may be to the overall benefit of social research, it could lead to a heavy emphasis on certain types of research, like, for instance, evaluative research, and on particular disciplines, such as health economics, to the possible exclusion or marginalization of other types of research and other disciplines (e.g. medical sociology, anthropology, political science).

Klein may be too optimistic in his assertion that as cracks appear in the consensus around health policy in the UK resulting from the introduction of market principles into the NHS, major opportunities will open up for researchers. Even if it were so, it is doubtful whether there exists sufficient research capacity to rise to the challenge without a fundamentally different approach to the way in which research is viewed, funded and organized. It is conceivable that the NHS Research and Development (R & D) strategy, introduced in 1991, will begin to address some of these structural concerns (Department of Health 1991). Indeed, there are signs that this may already be happening. These are considered further below. First, however, it is necessary to mention briefly other, more deep-seated impediments to the production and utilization of sound social research.

As Bulmer (1982: 115) has pointed out, there is a pervasive bias in British public life towards knowledge derived from the experience of the practitioner: 'he who does, knows'. This is not the place to explore these issues in detail, but if the position of social research is a reflection of a deeper anti-intellectualism in British public life, then the impediments to change are indeed considerable. By comparison with the USA, there is not the same enthusiasm for knowledge, for experimentation or for pilot projects which lend themselves to rigorous evaluation by an active and well-endowed research community harnessed to the cause (Hunter and Pollitt 1992). British pragmatism may also help to explain the recent conversion to, and seductive appeal of, 'quick fix' contract research and management consultancy. Solid, long-term social research is no longer viewed as attractive or fashionable – if it ever was. Managers and policy-makers want immediate definitive answers and solutions to urgent problems and are not prepared to defer gratification. Of course researchers are not entirely blameless in this neglect or outright dismissal of research. This dimension of the challenge is revisited in the next and final section.

But what about the NHS R & D incentive led by Michael Peckham and the task he has set himself, namely, the production of a 'comprehensive research and development strategy for the NHS' (Department of Health 1991)? Peckham's post – national director of R & D – is a new one and emerged from the DoH's response to the House of Lords Select Committee on Science and Technology which had produced a critical report on the government's priorities in medical research (House of Lords 1988). The DoH's response (Department of Health 1989) is replete with references to the importance of research, particularly in regard to the NHS reforms. Peckham maintains that the R & D initiative is probably 'the first comprehensive attempt to develop a national R & D infrastructure for health care .... [It] offers a unique opportunity to develop an overall view of basic and applied research in relation to health care and health priorities' (Peckham 1991: 371). Among the director's tasks are the following:

- advising the National Health Service Management Executive (NHSME) on priorities for NHS research and managing a programme of NHS research to meet identified needs, particularly research into the efficiency and effectiveness of health services
- ensuring that research information is widely disseminated and used by managers and practitioners to improve patient care.

(Department of Health 1989: para. 1.3.1)

In a specific reference to the NHS reforms, the DoH notes that health authorities, 'in concentrating on how to meet the health needs of their communities, may require local research to identify what those needs are and the effectiveness of services to meet them' (Department of Health, 1989: para. 2.14d.5).

This mention of research on health needs takes on added meaning and significance when set alongside the government's health strategy for England (Secretary of State for Health 1992). It stresses the importance of a clear strategic role for health authorities in maintaining and improving the health of their people and reaffirms the need to refocus attention on the broader public health issues which often go beyond the responsibilities of the NHS. The Secretary of State for Health asserts that research is essential to any strategy to improve health. The R & D strategy is therefore to be orientated towards attaining objectives within the key target areas and contributing new knowledge in other areas which will allow the health strategy to develop over time. The primary objective of the R & D strategy is 'to ensure that care in the NHS is based on high quality research relevant to improving the nation's health. In setting priorities for NHS R and D, opportunities for work which help the NHS increase its efficiency and promote health will have priority' (Secretary of State for Health 1992: para 5.6. 41–2).

Alongside the R & D strategy must be put the report of the task force on the strategy for research in nursing, midwifery and health visiting (Department of Health 1993a). This seeks to ensure that nursing research becomes a central part of the R & D strategy. A particular feature of the report is the need to improve research competence among nurses. Research in nursing should also be fully integrated within health services research.

Will the NHS R & D strategy assist the social research community in meeting the challenge posed by the health and social care reforms? And will it encourage health authorities to use and value research to greater effect? At this stage it is impossible to answer these questions. The strategy contains a number of elements intended to promote the value of research. For instance:

- Regional health authorities (RHAs) are required to prepare, publish, resource and implement (and be held to account for) R & D plans.
- National R & D priorities have been set.
- A central R & D committee has been established.
- Information systems on research outcomes for purchasers and providers of health care and for health policy and planning are being created.
- There is an emphasis on practical developments arising from research, and the prompt introduction of evaluated cost-effective developments in the NHS.

The objectives of the R & D strategy are set out in a summary of progress during its first two years (Department of Health 1993b). These are listed in Figure 1.2. The strategy places responsibility for its success on, among others, the 'research community' and its willingness and ability to take advantage of the opportunities opened up by the strategy.

Many, if not all, of the various elements which go to make up the

- To contribute to the health and well-being of the population through the conduct and application of relevant and high-quality R & D.
- To improve the scope, relevance and quality of R & D to inform policy and practice in health and social care.
- To facilitate the development of a knowledge-based NHS and encourage an evaluative culture within it.
- To harness the capacity of R & D, from basic science through to applied research, to address problems of national concern in health and social care.
- To ensure that the benefits of research are systematically and effectively translated into practice.
- To improve links between those involved in health and social care and research, whether as researchers, users of research findings or funders of research.

Figure 1.2 The objectives of the NHS Research and Development Strategy

strategy are laudable. Whether they succeed or not, at least an attempt is being made for the first time in the NHS to raise the importance and profile of health research (an important component of which is social research) and to ensure that any contribution research may have to make is made. Any progress in this area, however modest, is to be welcomed.

But there are dangers ahead and less reassuring aspects of the R & D strategy. The appointment of thirteen of the fourteen English regional directors of R & D, twelve of whom possess a medical background, offers clues as to how they may be expected to approach their task and as to their likely understanding and interpretation of social research. There is a real possibility that in the hands of individuals for whom social research is either little understood or dismissed as 'unscientific', or both, the research agenda will be biased towards biomedical research and to methodologies, notably randomized controlled trials, which fit such a bias (Hunter 1993b). If this happens, then investigator-led rather than problem-led research will remain dominant. The appointment in the autumn of 1993 of a social scientist as the deputy director of R&D nationally will go some way to correct this bias. However, the reduction of the number of regions to eight in April 1994 and their abolition in 1996 are creating uncertainty for the R&D strategy.

Other worrying aspects arising from the R & D strategy lurk within the research community itself. As the research agenda broadens to reflect a more holistic view of health as distinct from health care, then the 'departmentalitis' that is rife among the social science disciplines could become a more serious and divisive issue. It is doubtful if a centrally driven R & D strategy can prevent periodic outbreaks of factionalism within the research community. To some degree this structural defect has been recognized by Peckham. In 1991 he set up a review of the role of DoH-funded research units (Department of Health 1992b). In its controversial report, the review team recommended that the present number and structure of units should be replaced by a smaller number of larger interdisciplinary centres with a guaranteed ten-year period of funding. The existing system of centres is not seen to possess the necessary capacity or capability to provide the desired interdisciplinary environment. Not all researchers agree with this analysis or prescription. They argue that the case for change is unproven and that there is no evidence that large centres will be more productive, flexible or responsive than smaller ones (Maynard and Sheldon 1992).

At the nub of the dilemma posed by the R & D strategy and its likely impact are two key questions. Who sets the research agenda? Who defines the research questions to be addressed? Kelly (1990) goes some way towards considering these matters in the context of the World Health Organization's list of research priorities in its Health for All strategy (World Health Organization 1988). As he argues, agreement is required over which are the important research questions to investigate. This issue is closely related to who should make these decisions. The most obvious groups, as Kelly notes, are public health physicians and (social) epidemiologists. But they share a medically defined view of the world rather than a social or lay view. In similar vein, Levine and Sorenson (1983) maintain that health service policy-makers are more familiar with and amenable to the knowledge and technology of medicine than they are to the research findings and methods of the social and behavioural sciences. The challenge is to convince them of the error of their ways and to prevent the research agenda from being dominated by any one discipline or perspective. Most health and health policy issues do not occur as simple economic, psychological, sociological, epidemiological or clinical problems but as combinations of all of these. This point is well illustrated in Chapters 6 and 8 in this volume.

The problem is a fourfold one. It lies in part in many social researchers fighting shy of involvement in applied social research, for numerous reasons, including a desire to retain their objectivity, purity and integrity and thereby avoid contamination by a nasty world full of opportunists and self-seekers or, at best, misguided pragmatists and compromisers. Sometimes, these arguments are raised like a smokescreen behind which social scientists hide and protest. The fear of losing one's integrity may reside in a lack of confidence in one's ability to produce competent and useful research findings.

A second problem lies in researchers' own values, assumptions and preferences. It is nicely illustrated, possibly unintentionally, by Mays, when he observes that there are three distinctive research requirements:

> research to meet the political needs of Ministers and the DH; research which managers can use in running the NHS; and perhaps most important of all, independent, academic, strategic research which aims to improve understanding of health care and which will contribute ultimately to the more mundane interests of the first two areas.
> (Mays 1990: 31–2).

The use of the term 'mundane' is perhaps unfortunate and carries pejorative overtones which, regrettably, do little to promote good relations between researchers and policy-makers/managers.

The third problem, often a product of the other two, is the difficulty many practitioners, particularly managers and policy-makers, have in seeing the value of research and in being able to act upon it. In Britain at least, there is no culture of research in the delivery of health services or in their organization and management. Unlike some areas of medicine, research is not valued as a key aspect of professional development.

Finally, while it is essential for there to be proximity of the R & D function to the management process, there is a risk of research 'concentrating on issues of political significance and ignoring ones that are more important in relation to health care' (Cartwright 1992: 554). This could lead to a reluctance on the part of government to fund research that might yield uncomfortable evidence which might be seen to question or challenge current policy (Pollitt *et al.* 1990). Such a distortion of the research agenda is quite inimical to the research tradition.

Of course, none of these problems is new or a particular feature of the British health and social care reforms. However, these reforms give an added piquancy to them. The reasons for this concern the growing need for social research both on the impact of the reforms themselves and, increasingly, on the major topics of, *inter alia*, needs assessment, effective health care and the measurement of outcomes and user involvement in health care. The evolving policy agenda has unwittingly propelled social research into a prominent position, triggered by the paradigm shift we may be witnessing which puts health before health care services (Harrison *et al.* 1991). The public's health goes well beyond the NHS and embraces other areas of public policy that have an impact on the health of a population. Managers are groping cautiously, feeling exposed, vulnerable and inadequate in alien territory. Used to running things, buildings and people, those on the purchasing side of the purchaser–provider split are coming to realize that they need new skills and access to knowledge and data which had not hitherto been necessary. Social researchers have a window of opportunity available to them. Can they seize the initiative? Do they wish to? How?

SEIZING THE INITIATIVE

The fact that research is being done is not in dispute, although there may be legitimate concerns over its quality and thoroughness. A glance at the contents page of any recent health policy journal is indicative of the fertility of at least a sizeable body of researchers. But what is the outcome of all these labours? Refereed journal articles and impressive *curricula vitae*? Or the start of a genuine dialogue between researchers and those who fund and/or consume their labours?

The case for greater interaction among researchers, analysts, policy-makers and practitioners is not disputed and has been made repeatedly both in this country and in the USA (see, e.g., Hunter 1986, 1990; Shortell and Solomon 1982). Arguably, of particular importance in promoting a dialogue is the need to give closer attention to the *implementation* of health and social care policy. A similar concern was expressed some years ago by Smith (1986). He contrasted notions of 'middle-range' and 'micro' research issues with the 'macro' variables which shape policies and welfare systems. Of course 'big' research is needed, but the NHS reforms present a wealth of riches which are most appropriately addressed through middle-range and micro-modes of inquiry – albeit 'fraught with opportunity'.

Smith was articulating the case for a programme of social research on service delivery issues. He identified four topics or research streams (ibid.: 265):

1 the ideologies and impacts of frontline workers in service delivery
2 the role and impact of user perspectives on service delivery
3 the importance of inter-organizational relations and the overall system of care
4 the impact of organizational structures upon service delivery.

In the new world of purchasers (or enablers) and providers, contracts (or service agreements), medical audit, consumerism, total quality management and so on, these four topics, and the important contribution of social research to them, assume a renewed importance. As was pointed out earlier, the reforms have unleashed new behavioural responses and interpersonal dynamics which need to be documented in order to understand their operation and impact. The topics are germane to the issue of managing change, which is at the core of the reforms, particularly in their endeavour to shift the focus of attention from inputs into health and social services in favour of outcomes in terms of health impact. Research of both a middle-range and a micro variety 'serves as a useful corrective for the centralist and often simplistic perspectives of those who dominate policy-making networks' (Thompson 1986: 6).

Enhancing research utilization

Even on the rare occasions when social research is acknowledged as being of value, there remain problems at the interface between research findings and their use and implementation by management (Weir 1991). These are accepted by the DoH as being of some importance. The Research Management Division commissioned a report on the issue of research dissemination and ways of making better use of it (Richardson *et al.* 1990).

Weir, former chief scientist at the Scottish Office, has contrasted the position facing health-services research with that evident in clinical or biomedical research (Weir 1991). Whereas in the case of the latter it is the same group of professionals who undertake research and subsequently apply it, this is not so in respect of health services research, where very different groups carry out the research from those responsible for any subsequent implementation. Such a situation does not prevail in the USA where those who do research and those who implement it have a great deal in common (Fuchs 1990).

Social research can invariably be uncomfortable for policy-makers and practitioners alike. It can challenge cherished assumptions or appear destabilizing as ministers struggle to establish a new orthodoxy in the teeth of well-organized lobbies opposed to change. The sophisticated subtleties surrounding the successful management of change hold little appeal for ministers who are keen to leave their imprint on an area of policy. For them, quick, observable and dramatic change is demanded. Social research carries little appeal in such circumstances, for it seems only to add to the very confusion and complexity that reformers constantly seek to remove.

There are stratagems available to social researchers, and perhaps these need to be discussed more widely within the research community.

For example, researchers need (should) not restrict their search for impact on policy to the central arena. If policy is created locally as well as nationally (and the NHS reforms place a premium on local initiative even if it is tempered by the centrist political realities evident in many of the actions of the DoH/NHSME and Parliament), there may be considerable scope to influence local practice. Too often a 'top-down' model of the policy process is mirrored by a top-down model of the research process. Researchers feel obliged to influence the top wherever or whoever it is, although in fact their efforts may be better directed to the local level, where a great deal of policy-making goes on.

Second, researchers need to take not just research but also its dissemination seriously and to define clearly and target the audiences at whom it is aimed. This is the development part of R & D and is in danger of being overlooked. Getting R *into* D is a major challenge. Dissemination need not be only in written form but could take the form of workshops and so on which have a developmental or training dimension. If researchers cannot, or have no wish to, exercise or acquire these skills, then maybe there is a need for brokers to aid in the translation of policy research into both comprehensible and implementable forms. Perhaps it is a role for the new Schools of Public Health, and their variants, or for the dedicated NHS management education centres, which exist to provide training and development for public health doctors and managers and to carry out multidisciplinary research.

Third, and perhaps more difficult but also potentially more attractive at a time when virtually everyone in health and social care continues to struggle to interpret the various reforms and the meaning behind them, is the need to encourage managers to reflect upon their practice and to provide opportunities for them to do so (Schon 1983). The *craft* of management, as distinct from the *technique* of management, is predicated on the assumption that managing cannot be reduced to explicit rules and theories. As we move into uncharted waters as far as many of the NHS reforms are concerned, including the refocusing of the change agenda on the importance of health strategy with all its attendant uncertainties and puzzlement, then managers are likely to become more aware of the 'nonrational, intuitive artistry' (ibid.: 239) underpinning much management practice. Social research could assist in providing opportunities for managers to, in Schon's words, 'reflect-in-action'. This process seems particularly important in a situation of 'learning by doing' if the opportunities for policy and organizational learning are to be maximized.

CONCLUSION

The rediscovery of the value and importance of social research in the context of the NHS reforms and the R & D strategy is to be welcomed. Much social research is already under way to help enrich our knowledge and understanding of the NHS and associated reforms. Its value will, as this chapter has argued, largely be determined by the *level* at which it is carried out and by the ability of researchers to *empathize* with their organizational environment. Local studies aimed at changing local practices may achieve greater success than attempts to shift policy at the centre.

In maximizing the impact of social research and exploiting its potential to the full, social researchers may need to become more innovative and ingenious in engaging with policy-makers and managers in the hurly-burly of the political arena. Paradoxically, the opportunities for a dialogue are considerable because there are few guiding lights by which managers or others working in health and social care can steer their authorities into a safe haven. Social researchers may be able to help with the navigation provided policy-makers are truly committed to reaching a particular destination. The current politicization of health care reform, and the tactical manoeuvring it creates, are unhelpful in this respect.

For its part, the research infrastructure being established at national and regional levels arising from the R & D strategy must promote excellence and collaboration in research and not become an instrument for interference and collusion between researchers and policy-makers, with the former reduced to carrying out the latter's bidding and thereby losing their independence and credibility.

REFERENCES

Alford, R.R. (1975) *Health Care Politics*, Chicago: University of Chicago Press.

Bulmer, M. (1982) *The Uses of Social Research: Social Investigation in Public Policy-Making*, London: Allen & Unwin.

Cartwright, A. (1992) 'Health services research', *Journal of Epidemiology and Community Health* 46: 553–4.

Davey, B., and Popay, J. (1993) *Dilemmas in Health Care*, Milton Keynes: Open University Press.

Department of Health (1989) *Priorities in Medical Research*, Government Response to the Third Project of the House of Lords Select Committee on Science and Technology: 1987–8 Session, Cm 902, London: HMSO.

—— (1991) *Research for Health: A Research and Development Strategy for the NHS*, London: HMSO.

—— (1992a) *The Health of the Nation*, Cm 1986, London: HMSO.

—— (1992b) *Review of the Role of DH-Funded Research Units*, London: Department of Health.

—— (1993a) *Report of the Taskforce on the Strategy for Research in Nursing, Midwifery and Health Visiting*, London: Department of Health.

—— (1993b) *Research for Health*, London: Department of Health.

Evans, J.R. (1981) *Measurement and Management in Medicine and Health Services*, New York: Rockefeller Foundation.

Fuchs, B. (1990) *Medicare's Peer Review Organisations*, Washington, DC: Congressional Research Service Report to Congress.

Harrison, S., Hunter, D.J., Johnson, I., and Wistow, G. (1989) *Competing for Health: A Commentary on the NHS Review*, Leeds: Nuffield Institute for Health Services Studies, University of Leeds.

Harrison, S., Hunter, D.J., and Pollitt, C. (1990) *The Dynamics of British Health Policy* London: Unwin Hyman.

Harrison, S., Hunter, D.J., Johnston, I., Nicholson, N., Thunhurst, C., and Wistow, G. (1991) *Health before Health Care*, London: Institute for Public Policy Research.

Harrison, S., Hunter, D.J., Marnoch, G., and Pollitt, C. (1992) *Just Managing: Power and Culture in the NHS*, Basingstoke: Macmillan.

House of Lords (1988) 'Priorities in medical research', Select Committee on Science and Technology Session 1987–88 Third Report, HL Paper 54, London: HMSO.

Hunter, D.J. (1986) *Managing the NHS in Scotland: Review and Assessment of Research Needs*, Scottish Health Service Studies 45, Edinburgh: Scottish Home and Health Department.

—— (1988) 'The impact of research on restructuring the British NHS', *The Journal of Health Administration Education* 6, 3: 537–53.

—— (1990) 'Organising and managing health care: a challenge for medical sociology', in Cunningham-Burley, S. and McKeganey, N.P. eds, *Readings in Medical Sociology*, London: Tavistock/Routledge.

—— (1993a) 'The internal market: the shifting agenda', in Tilley, I. ed., *Managing the Internal Market*, London: Paul Chapman.

—— (1993b) 'Let's hear it for R and D', *Health Service Journal*, 15 April: 17.

Hunter, D.J., and Pollitt, C. (1992) 'Developments in health services research: perspectives from Britain and the United States', *Journal of Public Health Medicine* 14, 2: 164–8.

Kelly, M. (1990) 'The role of research in the new public health', *Critical Public Health* 3: 4–9.

Klein, R. (1990) 'Research, policy and the NHS', *Journal of Health Politics, Policy and Law* 15, 3: 501–23.

Levine, S., and Sorenson, J.R. (1983) 'Medical sociology and health administration', *The Journal of Health Administration Education* 1 4: 343–82.

Mawhinney, B., and Nichol, D. (1993) *Purchasing for Health*, London: National Health Service Management Executive.

Maynard, A., and Sheldon, T. (1992) 'Reforming the Department of Health's Research and Development policy: from the devil to the deep blue sea?', *British Medical Journal* 305: 1209–10.

Mays, N. (1990) 'Clout and credibility? The new director of research and development in the department of health', *Critical Public Health* 3: 26–32.

Peckham, M. (1991) 'Research and Development for the NHS', *The Lancet* 338: 367–71.

Pole, J.E. (1966) *Medicine and Politics*, London: Pitman Medical.

Pollitt, C., Harrison, S., Hunter, D.J., and Marnoch, G. (1990) 'No hiding place: on the discomforts of researching the contemporary policy process', *Journal of Social Policy*, 19, 2: 169–90.

Richardson, A., Jackson, C., and Sykes, W. (1990) *Taking Research Seriously*, London: HMSO.

Schon, D.A. (1983) *The Reflective Practitioner: How Professionals Think in Action*, New York: Basic Books.

Secretaries of State for Health, Social Security, Wales and Scotland (1989) *Caring for People*, Cm 846, London: HMSO.

Secretaries of State for Health, Wales, Northern Ireland and Scotland (1989) *Working for Patients*, Cm 555, London: HMSO.

Shortell, S.M., and Solomon, M.A. (1982) 'Improving health care policy research', *Journal of Health Politics, Policy and Law* 6, 4: 684–702.

Smith, G. (1986) 'Service delivery issues', *The Quarterly Journal of Social Affairs* 2, 3: 265–83.

Stowe, K. (1989) *On Caring for the National Health*, London: Nuffield Provincial Hospitals Trust.

Thompson, F.J. (1986) 'The health policy context', in Hill, C.E. ed., *Current Health Policy Issues and Alternatives: An Applied Social Science Perspective* Athens, Ga: University of Georgia Press.

Weir, R. (1991) 'Research in public health: who says, who does, who cares?', Faculty of Public Health Medicine, Queen Elizabeth the Queen Mother Annual Lecture, Royal College of Physicians of London (unpublished lecture, delivered 30 January).

World Health Organization (1988) *Priority Research for Health for All*, Copenhagen: World Health Organization.

Chapter 2

The place of research in a consumer-led system of health care

Gilbert Smith, Jennie Popay and Gareth Williams

INTRODUCTION

Although there is a widespread tendency amongst commentators to refer to the National Health Service (NHS) reforms as if they had happened already, it still may be premature to take that stance. Many of the most fundamental changes will take some time to work through the system. It is true that changes to administrative and some policy-making mechanisms have been introduced, following legislation, with a degree of speed and determination that has not always characterized public-sector planning in the UK. But other aspects of this latest 'reorganization of the NHS' are taking a little longer.

For example, purchasing authorities have been reined in during the first two years of their operations. They have largely been confined to the task of arranging for a service similar to that provided previously – but within the new structure. The Minister for Health has now turned his attention to these new strategic authorities, arguing in April 1993 that 'from now on the NHS needs to be a purchaser driven organisation . . . purchasers have a responsibility to force the pace of change' (Mawhinney 1993: 10, 12). However, only in the years ahead will we see whether aggressive and imaginative purchasing strategies can significantly alter patterns of care. They must in many cases do this within the context of zero-sum alterations in the distribution of resources within and between services. The alternative is the 'rising tide' approach, which produces changes only by assigning to new priorities any growth finance available. But, in the short term at least, many purchasing authorities will see little if any growth monies. The resources available to them are being strongly influenced by the introduction of a new system of capitation funding in parallel with the other NHS reforms in 1991 (Department of Health 1989). This is producing winners and losers on the financial front with profound implications for the purchasing process. Finally, we have yet to see how free NHS trust managers will really be in questions of charges, raising capital, specialization of services, and other matters. It is, however, evident that the reforms are fuelling a rationalization of acute sector services – particularly, but not exclusively, in the big cities.

So there are many issues outstanding. Yet amidst them there is one question that is particularly important. It is this. What will it take to allow public health data on health needs, health care outputs, and the efficiency and efficacy of health care interventions to *drive* the system?

There is much agreement that up to now the patterns of provision in the NHS have been heavily *provider*-led. Left-wing social scientists of the 1960s, in their criticisms of professional dominance (Illich 1976; Navarro 1976), and right-of-centre politicians of the 1980s, in their advocacy of the interests of the consumer, are at one on that point. Many advocates of the NHS reforms now argue that market forces shall be the new determinants of developments and of both high and low priorities. But the early period of the reforms has shown two things rather clearly. The idea of health care being like any other marketable commodity is politically very unpopular, and the market in health care is in any case at most only a 'quasi-market'. There are too many restrictions for the operation of true market forces to apply in this setting.

That is why the alternative possibility – that of change being driven by public-health data – is potentially so important. This view is now being advocated by the politicians steering the reforms. In an important speech on 'The Vision of Purchasing' in April 1993, for example, Brian Mawhinney, Minister for Health argued:

> Information and intelligence are the life-blood of purchasers. Their decisions must be based on sound evidence about health needs, clinical and cost-effectiveness and costs and prices . . . . there is no substitute for detailed local investigations and these should underpin all major purchasing decisions.
>
> (Mawhinney 1993: 18)

On the other hand there are those who would argue that to take seriously the possibility of 'knowledge-based' purchasing is itself over-rationalistic or just simply naive.

RESEARCH AND THE NHS REFORMS

These introductory comments give some indication of just why it is that research is so crucial in relation to the current round of NHS reforms. In the previous chapter, David Hunter rightly noted that, whatever the reaction to the merits or otherwise of the NHS reforms, there can be no doubt at all that they represent a most interesting challenge to the social-science community.

Of course, the relationship between social research and social policy is *always* important, but in the past that research has generally taken one, or both, of two forms. First, social research has investigated the presumptions upon which a particular policy innovation is predicated. Thus, for example, recent changes in the education system have made assumptions about the way in which parental choice is exercised in relation to children's education. Similarly, Department of Health initiatives to reduce waiting-lists for health care and lengths of patient waiting-times make presumptions about the meaning of waiting-list data. Generally, the assumptions underlying policy are open to empirical study through social research. Research on waiting-lists, for instance, has demonstrated their complexity and the misguided nature of policy-makers' assumptions in this area (Pope 1991).

Second, research has often performed an evaluative function. Although the design of evaluation research presents many methodological and conceptual difficulties, in a variety of ways research can try to give guidance on whether or not the policy has been a 'successful' one in relation to its declared objectives. Do parents experience greater choice of schools for their children? Is medical treatment provided with less delay? These questions are not quite as straightforward as they may at first appear, but they are researchable.

However, in the case of the 1991 NHS reforms the potential relationship between policy and research is neither of these two kinds. Here social-science data are cast in such a role that they are an integral part of the policy change. It is a fundamental component of the policy initiative that purchasing authorities shall assess the needs of the population for which they are responsible and base their purchasing of health care upon such an assessment (National Health Service Management Executive 1991; Mawhinney 1993). Research in general, and social research in particular, is not thus, as it were, an 'optional extra'. As the national Director of Research and Development recently argued, 'the NHS cannot do without research and development' (Smith 1993: 1407). Anything approaching a full implementation of the radical intentions of the NHS reforms simply will not take place without it. Thus the generation and effective use of more and better data is a critical factor in what David Hunter describes in his chapter as the 'shift in power relations between the principal actors, notably doctors and managers' (see also Flynn 1992).

Key questions

Shifts in power relations do not take place spontaneously, however, so there is more to the implementation of the NHS reforms than the simple rational application of a body of social science data. Much depends on the answers to some key questions.

First, are politicians and policy-makers at central government level really prepared for the changes that could follow in the wake of the reforms that they have brought about, or will the exercise of even limited market forces and changed patterns of influence produce a degree of destabilization in health care that proves politically unacceptable? Second, and likewise, have the radical changes that could follow in the wake of a complete departure from the historic base of district funding that is entailed in capitation funding been fully accepted? Third, is the medical profession really prepared to accept a position of influence in the NHS that is substantially different from that which it has consistently occupied since 1948? Finally, will purchasing authorities be able to develop sufficient influence in relation to NHS trusts and other provider units to be able to exert genuine influence over the nature and quality of care in a 'managed market'?

NECESSARY AND SUFFICIENT CONDITIONS FOR CHANGE

The answer to these questions, and indeed the future success of purchasing authorities as 'the engines for improving NHS performance' (Nichols 1993: 57), will depend upon a variety of developments, the future direction of which is uncertain at the moment. The NHS reforms are indeed uncharted waters, the political arena is highly volatile, and the processes of political and organizational learning are unpredictable. Within this turmoil the following six key developments will be significant.

Organizational developments

The development of the purchaser–provider relationship in the NHS reforms lies at the heart of many of the changes. Both major political parties have made it clear that they expect the purchaser–provider relationship now to be a permanent feature of the NHS. The process of providing a majority of services through trusts has proceeded quickly, and the government's expectation is that by April 1994 95 per cent of NHS hospitals and community health service provision will have trust status and one in three patients will be registered with fundholding general practitioners (GPs). The form that competition will take will rest heavily upon whether or not trusts are able to create a monopoly in supply in their areas, and whether or not purchasing authorities will be prepared to put their traditional suppliers of services at risk by buying cheaper and better services from other trusts. Variations in geographical context will also be important in determining how realistic it will be for purchasers to choose between providers.

Financial developments

Capitation funding, introduced in 1991 alongside the reforms to determine the distribution of resources at regional and district levels, is crucial if purchasers are to be able to build their care strategies on a new balance between needs and resources, rather than just make incremental changes to a historical base. The new capitation funding system means that since 1992/3 regional and district health authorities have received NHS funds on the basis of the relative size and composition of their resident populations, weighted for selected factors. (There are also development monies made available against bids each year, but these represent a very small proportion of district budgets.)

A form of capitation funding existed before 1991. In 1976, for example, the Resource Allocation Working Party (RAWP) set target funding for regions on the basis of their resident populations, weighted for age, sex and mortality and allowing for patient flows across boundaries (Department of Health and Social Security 1976). This system did begin to change – albeit slowly – the historical pattern of allocation, which was strongly shaped by the geographical spreads of hospital care and dominated by large teaching hospitals. Disparities between regions reduced from a 27 per cent range between the best-off and the worst-off in 1977/8 (Winyard 1981) to 4 per cent in 1986/7 (Mays and Bevan 1987). There was, however, little change below regional level.

The 1991 reforms have speeded up the move towards capitation funding overall, but especially at sub-regional level. This has predictably generated a vigorous debate about the validity and justice of the formulas now being used to weight population figures (Sheldon *et al.* 1993; Raftery 1993). Existing formulas have resulted in some rural areas and seaside resorts gaining significantly at the expense of inner-city areas. Formula funding brings to an end the continuous process of 'bidding' for resources; but, of course, that much more is dependent on the construction of the formula in the first place.

One approach to the practical but also political problems created by the 'winners' and 'losers' scenario is to adopt the 'rising tide' approach mentioned earlier. This presumes that growth monies will become available and that these will be used to bring 'underfunded' districts up to their 'target'. But there are two problems in this approach. First, there is the danger of recreating all the problems associated with the slow movement towards the old RAWP targets – a position from which it was precisely intended the NHS reforms should move away. Second, this approach is not consistent with the objective of encouraging sensible prioritization in resource allocation which should be able to function even in the context of level funding.

Clearly, much more work needs to be undertaken on the formula itself and on the relative health-related costs of different population groups – notably the elderly. Recent research into the purchasing process suggests that the financial state of purchasing organizations is a crucial factor in their ability to change services:

> There were plenty of examples of how 'new monies' either from development funds or from relative growth related to weighted capitation was influencing the shape of health services . . . where there was no new money, and the development budget was effectively being used as a contingency fund against mishaps . . . the emphasis was much more on containing a potentially explosive situation than being the architect of change . . . the somewhat arbitrary weighted capitation formula is the single most important influence upon the health and vitality of purchasing.
>
> (Freemantle *et al.* 1993: 32–3)

Technical and managerial developments

There are certain technical and managerial developments in the administration of purchasing-authority business which are important and which are closely linked. Most purchasing authorities will probably be structured internally in a not dissimilar way. They will have directorates of Finance, Public Health, Quality Assurance and Consumer Affairs, Information, Planning and Contracting. The titles and combinations of functions may differ somewhat but there is unlikely to be a great deal of variation.

A key question is whether or not they can arrange their business so as to base decisions on a common data set. In principle such a requirement looks obvious and straightforward. In practice it will not be easy to achieve. But for a purchasing strategy to determine effective patterns of care, financial information, good public health data on health care needs, data that monitor and inform the contracting process, quality and consumer feedback data, and demographic and other data to set the medium- and long-term planning context, must all be integrated into a single package and used as a common base by all directorates. Technically, in employing the right information systems, and managerially, in setting up the right working relationships and day-to-day office practices, this will be difficult. As Ong in Chapter 4 and Williams and Popay in Chapter 6 argue, these systems will also have to be complemented by qualitative information from a range of sources, and this will bring other difficulties. Finally, it is not self-evident that the new purchasing authorities, with their small staffing levels, will have the capacity to deal with the complex intelligence systems they will require.

Political developments

It is often argued by opponents of the NHS reforms that they have been devised in response to political dogma and are being forced through at a pace which is unreasonably rapid. Other commentators might well note that there are sections of the map of what the future health service might look like which have still to be charted. Much will depend on political developments.

Any Conservative government is aware that market forces, once unleashed, do not always produce changes which are popular, even with those who support the reforms in general. There is already evidence that purchasers in some regions are coming under pressure to support local units where they are the major purchasers rather than put them at risk of closure by 'buying' elsewhere at lower costs or greater effectiveness (Freemantle *et al.* 1993). Any future Labour government will have to confront the problem of a health service always being 'underfunded' (because of near-unlimited demand on limited funds). It will also have the difficulty of implementing new priorities where these were opposed by the weight of the medical profession, unless some alternative driving force is poured into the vacuum that is otherwise filled by market forces or professional dominance.

Professional developments

We have already mentioned on several occasions the importance of the role of the medical profession in deciding the future course of the NHS reforms. Hitherto, public health has not been a high-status specialty within medicine. However, it is clear that the 'new public health' has a major role to play, and much will depend upon whether or not it can achieve a position of prestige from which to exert influence. Recent commentators remain to be convinced that public health medicine in particular has the capacity to fulfil this role, and the importance of a multidisciplinary endeavour is increasingly recognized (Alderslade and Hunter 1992). It has also been argued that the medical profession may yet reassert its authority over health care, and with it the traditional provider focus may return centre-stage (Hunter 1992).

Intellectual developments

A high proportion of the developments so far discussed are dependent on the outcome of political and social processes. There is therefore more to change than the application of new knowledge. Nevertheless, certain intellectual developments could have a crucial influence on the answers to the four key questions posed earlier.

It will be vital for the social science of health-needs assessment to progress rapidly. Perhaps the comparison is a little dramatic, but the reform of the NHS is not unlike the declared intent to land a man (or woman) on the moon without having invented the rocket to carry them there. Many methodological and conceptual problems remain to be solved, and it will be difficult for social science data to drive the system until they are. Some of these problems are discussed in the chapter that follows, and the magnitude of the challenge for social science and indeed other disciplines is clearly illustrated. The somewhat rudimentary state of the needs-assessment process within most purchasing authorities is clear. Two comments made to Nick Freemantle and his colleagues (1993) during their recent research illustrate this point: '[it's] about time we gave up on this notion of needs assessment . . . it's a joke . . . we should be honest and admit it' (Public Health Medicine Consultant); 'I leave all that health needs nonsense to public health . . . it's irrelevant' (Director of Contracts).

CONCLUSION

So far as the NHS reforms are concerned, social research and health policy are now locked together. They are locked together by the very nature of the changes that have been set in train. So the question to ask is not the usual one of 'Does social science have a contribution to make?' If it does not, then the reforms will have been profoundly mistaken in their conception. The question is: 'What will it take to allow social research to fulfil that role which is inherent in the attempt to move from a provider-led to a purchaser-led system of health care?'

Several developments – organizational, financial, technical, managerial, political, professional and intellectual – will be crucial in ensuring that the place of research in a consumer-led system of health care is a constructive one. If it is not constructive, then this will not only represent a failure for the research community. The NHS reforms will also have failed in their attempt to influence the movement of resources and patterns of care from a historic case to one which demonstrably responds to the population's health care needs.

REFERENCES

Alderslade, R., and Hunter, D. (1992) 'Forward march: a green light for public health management', *Health Service Journal* 102, 5294: 22–3.

Department of Health (1989) *Funding and Contracts for Hospital Services*, Working For Patient Working Paper 2, London: HMSO.

Department of Health and Social Security (1976) *Resource Allocation Working Party Report*, London: HMSO.

Flynn, R. (1992) *Structures of Power and Control in Health Management*, London: Routledge.

Freemantle, N., Watts, I., and Mason, J. (1993) 'Talking shop', *Health Service Journal* 103, 5357: 31–3.

Hunter, D. (1992) 'Doctors as managers: poachers turned gamekeepers? *Social Science & Medicine* 35, 4: 557–66.

Illich, I. (1976) *Limits to Medicine*, New York: Marion Boyars.

Mawhinney, B. (1993) 'The vision for purchasing', in Mawhinney, B., and Nichols, D. *Purchasing for Health: A Framework for Action*, Leeds: National Health Service Management Executive.

Mays, N., and Bevan, G. (1987) *Resource Allocation in the Health Service: A Review of the Resource Allocation Working Party*, London: Bedford Press.

National Health Service Management Executive (1991) *Assessing Health Care Needs: A DHA Project Discussion Paper*, London: HMSO.

Navarro, V. (1976) *Medicine under Capitalism*, New York: Prodist.

Nichols, D. (1993) 'Reaping the benefits', in Mawhinney, B., and Nichols, D. *Purchasing for Health: A Framework for Action*, Leeds: National Health Service Management Executive.

Pope, C. (1991) 'Trouble in store: some thoughts on the management of waiting lists', *Sociology of Health and Illness* 13, 2: 193–212.

Raftery, J. (1993) 'Capitation funding: population, age and mortality adjustments for regional and district health authorities in England', *British Medical Journal* 307: 112–24.

Sheldon, T., Davey-Smith, G., and Bevan, G. (1993) 'Weighting in the dark; resource allocation in the new NHS', *British Medical Journal* 306: 835–9.
Smith, R. (1993) 'Filling the lacuna between research and practice: an interview with Michael Peckham', *British Medical Journal* 307: 1407.
Winyard, P. (1981) 'RAWP – new injustice for old', *British Medical Journal* 286: 112.

Part II

The theory and methods of needs assessment

Chapter 3

The conceptualization and measurement of need

A social policy perspective

Jonathan Bradshaw

> You can't always get what you want
> you can't always get what you want
> you can't always get what you want
> but if you try sometime
> you might find
> you get what you need!
>
> (Michael Jagger circa 1967)

INTRODUCTION

Need is a modern concept. I understand that the word has no equivalent in ancient Greek or Latin. In fact it was not used very widely in the context of the social life of England until after the Second World War. The Poor Law was concerned with deserts, motives, destitution, obligations, eligibility and, rarely, rights. In his research around the turn of the century, the social researcher and commentator Seebohm Rowntree (1901) was preoccupied with primary and secondary poverty and minimum subsistence income. In his plans for the British Welfare State, Beveridge (Cmnd 6404 1942) did not talk about needs; he talked about 'Giant Evils'. There is a Ph.D. for an historical lexicographer in tracing how this word has grown in prominence today. As an idea with meaning in social science it (still) leaves a great deal to be desired.

Twenty-five years ago I wrote a paper which attempted to present a taxonomy of social need (Bradshaw 1972). For this chapter I was originally asked to dust off the ideas in that article and direct them at the subject of health needs. However, I do not believe that this is a worthwhile thing to do. Instead, I wish to argue that the concept of need has always been too imprecise, too complex, too contentious to be a useful target for policy. Also (and therefore) it has serious limitations as an epidemiological identifier and as a basis for evaluating the performance of policies. I shall review briefly the work of philosophers who have struggled with the notion of categorical need but failed, I think, to produce a solution that helps the policy-maker and policy-analyst. I shall refer to the work of economists who have abandoned the search for a meaning of need independent of the resources that are available. I shall argue that the use of the concept of need by Thatcherite politicians has further discredited need as an idea with special imperative for action. Finally, I shall discuss the meanings given to the concept of health needs. If we are to accept a social definition of health needs, then I argue that, instead of need, a more appropriate target for health and other public policy (but not perhaps the health service), one that avoids the problem of need, and that has been neglected if not covered up during the last decade, is inequality.

THE CONCEPT OF NEED

The classification of social need that I devised (so long ago) was developed in a less harsh world, as part of a Master's thesis. There was no practical intent, other than to help to sort out what the word 'need' meant when applied to the social needs of people aged over 80 (the subject of the thesis). I distinguished between four different types of need:

1 *Normative need* is defined by experts, professionals, doctors, policy-makers, and so on. Often a desirable standard is laid down and compared with the standard that actually exists.
2 *Felt need* is want, desire or subjective views of need which may or may not become expressed need.
3 *Expressed need* is demand or felt need turned into action.
4 *Comparative need*, which I did not describe very well, has to do with equity.

In the discussion of the original classification, I suggested that when we describe someone as being 'in need' we have in mind some permutation of these four categories of need. In fact conceptually (allowing for the fact that expressed need cannot exist without felt need) there are ten permutations of need and it is possible to think up examples that represent each permutation. The taxonomy was never presented as a way of ranking the priority of needs. It is probable that in any particular case *real* need would exist when each of the four elements was present at the same time. However, for example, some normative needs might be very urgent and not felt or expressed. Certainly need (comparative) can exist in one area or group at the same time as not being felt, expressed or recognized as a need normatively. The most that could be claimed for the taxonomy was that it was helpful for undergraduate students, and that those seeking to evaluate the extent to which services meet needs or to assess needs in the community might have found it useful to differentiate between the different types of need.

Since all this was published there has been added a vast literature on need. Included among it have been some good critical reviews of my taxonomy. For example, Clayton (1983) pointed out that there could be, and often is, more than one judgement about normative need and that comparative need is likely to be the consequence of the application of a normative judgement on need by a different person and/or at a different time and/or in a different place. The taxonomy has been employed as an *aide-mémoire* or a structure of thinking for a variety of studies of need, including the needs of local communities (Ife 1980), legal need (Robertson 1991), housing need (Clayton 1983) and need for help from the Social Fund (Huby and Dix 1992).

Spek (1972) has developed an alternative classification for health needs in which needs are judged by three parties, society, experts and individuals, and needs are assessed by answering two questions: 'Is the individual sick?' and 'Is the individual in need of public care?' More recently, the National Health Service (NHS) reforms introduced at the beginning of the 1990s emphasized the assessment of health needs to inform the strategic thinking of the new purchasing health authorities and spawned a new set of studies in the health field (see, for example, Chapters 4 and 6 for a discussion of some of this work).

Also since my original work appeared an enormous literature on need has been published that has developed understanding of the concept very considerably. Strong contributions to this literature have come particularly from philosophers and economists.

Philosophers

Moral philosophers have, *inter alia*, argued about the distinction between instrumental and categorical need, explored the moral basis of need and helped us to distinguish between need and two other concepts – desire and interest. There has been a debate, partly philosophical and partly socio-political, about whether basic, fundamental or categorical needs exist or whether need is (merely) a relative concept and/or instrumental (see Sen 1981; Townsend 1979). For a substantial review of this literature, see Doyal and Gough (1991). It has been argued (Wiggins 1987; Megone 1992) that needs which have to be fulfilled in order for a person to develop properly as a human being can be classed as categorical needs. These needs, which a human cannot do without, are overriding and include health, nutrition and shelter. They are overriding because they are inherent to the need itself and our nature as human beings.

I am prepared to accept these arguments in principle, although some do not (Barry 1965) and others have added to the list of categorical human needs particular autonomy or the capacity or freedom to choose (Doyal and Gough 1991). However, in relating these arguments to policy they still leave us somewhat bereft. What level of health, nutrition and shelter is required? At what level of human development are we aiming? If the answers to those questions are couched in relative terms, then what guidance are we given about our moral obligations collectively or individually to meet needs?

Economists

Economists (in particular Williams 1978; 1992) seek to abandon the language of 'needology' and introduce instead the language of priorities. Here the questions are not what need is and who is in need but who is to have first claim on limited resources and who is to judge that claim? What are the trade-offs?

> We are in the business of making judgements about the relative values of different potential benefits to different potential beneficiaries, and we are not helped in that difficult intellectual and political task by thought-stopping terms like 'need' which invite 'on–off' thinking rather than 'more–less' thinking.
>
> (Williams 1992: 62)

Inevitably this language of choice takes us towards an instrumental view of needs because it is the relationship between the means and the ends, and the criteria for judging that relationship, that matter. Thus Culyer (1992) suggests that the task of the social scientist is to establish what are the most efficient means of meeting certain ends. Which needs should be met first for an end to be most cost-effectively achieved?

Politicians

Policy-makers have become more and more obsessed with need. Indeed the 1980s could be described as the decade of need. A government committed to rolling back the boundaries of the State, reducing public expenditure and cutting taxation has sought to achieve these objectives by 'concentrating help where it is needed most'. In a whole number of policy areas, in order to implement cuts (and minimize their political costs) some criterion or other has had to be established to identify *real* need as opposed to other types of need. On a number of occasions ministers have attempted to deal with the problem of defining *real* need by arguing it out of existence. Thus, for example, the unfortunate John Moore, when Secretary of State for Social Services, made a speech (11 May 1989) announcing the 'end of the line' for poverty. It was really only inequality, he said, and he argued that those who expressed concern about poverty were either politically motivated, or motivated by envy. In the social security field this ideology has resulted in the withdrawal of Income Support for young people, cuts in benefit levels for the unemployed, the freezing of Child Benefit, a massive extension of means-testing and the reintroduction of discretionary decision-making in the Social Fund. In the health field, needs assessment has been advocated as a means of containing the growth of health costs (as well as hopefully increasing the cost-effectiveness of the expenditure).

What *real* need means in any different policy area has of course varied. The case of the Social Fund is a good example of the tangle into which the concept of need has fallen. Need is what claimants ask for – but only if they meet the criteria in the Act and regulations, if they belong to one of the priority groups listed in the guidance to Social Fund officers, if the item they ask for is also considered a priority in that guidance, if the Social Fund officer recognizes all this, and then only if there is money left in the local office budget. If there is no money in the budget, then however high the priority of the claimant and the item requested, it is not need. The Social Fund is all dressed up in the language of need – Social Fund officers are said to be 'meeting need'; the objective of the social fund is to meet needs which cannot be met out of the scale rates of benefit; the objective of research is to evaluate whether needs are being met. In fact the word 'need' has become a smoke-screen to hide the true intention of policy, to camouflage policies which in their intention and effect have the explicit purpose of increasing inequalities. If the word 'need' ever had any analytical purpose in the social sciences, it has been cynically adulterated in the last ten or so years.

HEALTH NEEDS

What is health need? To seek to answer that question we have to establish some understanding of what health is. There are broadly two models of health, and each has rather different consequences for the understanding of health needs and their implications for health and social policy.

The medical model views health as the absence of clinically ascertainable disease (Helman 1981). Need in this context would be the presence of disease which is treatable successfully. The emphasis is on cure rather than prevention, disease rather than the promotion of health and welfare, and the treatment of the individual rather than of social conditions. This model is reflected in the practice and structures of medicine in society, in the emphasis given to the treatment of specific conditions, in the priority accorded to acute specialist medicine, in the assessment of health needs by the use of waiting-lists for treatment and in the use of inputs as outputs such as the number of operations performed or patients treated per bed.

The alternative is the social model of health commonly associated with the World Health Organization (WHO) definition: 'a state of complete physical, mental and social well-being and not merely the absence of disease or infirmity'. This has been complemented by the more recent definition:

> the extent to which an individual or group is able, on the one hand, to realise aspirations and satisfy needs and on the other hand, to change or cope with the environment. Health is therefore seen as resources for every day life, not the objective of living: it is a positive concept emphasising social and personal resources as well as physical capacities.
>
> (World Health Organization 1985)

As well as curative medicine this model emphasizes prevention, recovery and rehabilitation. It focuses on the interaction between health and the social structure. Thus it emphasizes the impact of disadvantage and inequalities. Need is not an absolute state, not just an untreated condition, not just an impairment or a disability, but also an absence of well-being or quality of life. It is a handicap that is socially defined. Meeting need is not the treatment of disease but whether the quality of life is enhanced as a result. For the most efficient meeting of health needs we may need to look beyond improvements in detection, diagnosis, cure, medical delivery and even prevention and health education, to changes in the social structure itself – to changes in the material conditions in which people live and the life-chances they have available to them. To identify ill-health we may have to have recourse to other methods than the diagnostic skills of medical practitioners. Self-reports – the experience, assessments and subjective feelings of people (their felt needs) – have greater importance and validity. The kind of measures (discussed in Chapter 10 by Ray Fitzpatrick) that incorporate physical, social and emotional factors and psycho-social well-being are of increasing usefulness. Indeed, there is growing evidence that measures of this type are powerful predictors of subsequent mortality (Kaplan and Kotler 1985).

PROBLEMS WITH HEALTH NEEDS

There is a variety of problems associated with the social definition of health as the determinant of health needs and of priorities for the NHS.

First, there is the argument that the agenda for the NHS would become hopelessly ambitious if it aimed to deal with the wider definition of health. This kind of response was illustrated by the government's reaction to the Black Report on inequalities in health in 1980 (Black *et al.* 1988). Instead of being properly printed and published, 260 duplicated copies were slipped out without a press release on the Friday before August Bank Holiday with a curt dismissal from Patrick Jenkin to the effect that: 'the report's recommendations . . . are quite unreasonable in the present or any foreseeable economic circumstances, quite apart from any judgement that may be formed of the effectiveness of such expenditure in dealing with the problems identified' (ibid.: 4). He was speaking as Minister of Health, but health professionals may feel justified in arguing that even if the causes of illness lie in the social structure, they cannot, with the resources at their disposal, do anything about it.

Second, there is the argument that the association between poverty and ill-health is not sufficiently well understood for effective interventions to be planned. Thus, for example, although we know that poor maternal diet is associated with low birth-weights, we do not know what social policy would be an effective response to the problem of poor maternal diets. Or, to take another example, we know that damp houses create fungus spores which cause respiratory disease, but do we know how to ensure that houses are not damp?

Third, there is the argument that ill-health is not entirely the consequence of structural factors which might be adapted by social policy. It also has something to do with variations in the innate characteristics and capacities of populations – the most obvious example of this is the class variation in the prevalence of congenital defects. It also has something to do with variations in behaviour. Thus the poor may be more likely to be unhealthy because they eat the wrong food, smoke more (but drink less), do not bring themselves to maternity services or their children for immunization, are more liable to marital breakdown or out-of-wedlock births with their attendant health risks. These behaviourial causes of ill-health were emphasized in *The Health of the Nation* (Department of Health 1992), but the fact that they exist does not mean that they are impervious to influence or change. Additionally, as research has demonstrated, individual behaviour is strongly linked to the social and material circumstances in which people live (Graham 1987).

Fourth, inequalities in health, given their socio-structural determinants, seem impervious to change. The continued existence of widespread inequalities in health forty years after the establishment of the NHS is taken as an indication of its inability to tackle inequalities in health. After all, was it not one of the principal objectives of the NHS to equalize access by providing health care free at the point of need?

There is in fact a good deal of disagreement about the distributional consequences of health expenditure. Le Grand (1982) estimated that after controlling for the higher morbidity among the lower classes, health expenditure was regressive. Expenditure per ill person was 40 per cent higher in the top class than the bottom class. These findings have been explored by others who have queried the value of self-reported morbidity data (which was used to control for variations in need), not least because self-reported morbidity has been increasing among the better-off (Le Grand 1991; O'Donnell and Propper 1989).

So there is doubt about whether the distributional effects of health spending are as bad as has been estimated. Furthermore, many of the mechanisms that lead to regressive outcomes for health spending are known about and can be dealt with. They include inequities in the spatial distribution of spending, inequities in the sector distribution of spending (acute vs prevention), greater propensity to utilize health services among the middle classes owing to confidence, knowledge and articulateness, and barriers to access for people in the lower classes, including their reliance on public transport.

HEALTH INEQUALITIES

There is disagreement in the literature about whether inequalities in health are increasing or diminishing. This is not surprising given the enormous methodological problems involved in exploring the issue. These include problems with the indicators of health, particularly morbidity, that are available. However, the main problem has been to do with the indicators of stratification, particularly the most common one, social class. Because of changes in the class distribution over time, because of changes in family form, particularly the increased prevalence of lone parents and dual-worker families, social class based on the employment of the head of the household is an increasingly unsatisfactory indicator of stratification over time. As an alternative Illsley and Le Grand (1987) have explored differences between the ages at which people die by a variety of inequality measures and found a sharp decline in the inequalities. They have also looked at regional variations in age-specific death-rates and found sharp falls in variation since 1931, except for men aged 45 and 64.

Whatever the trends over time, inequalities in health remain very wide. The rate of still births, infant mortality and the standardized mortality rate of adults is in each case twice as high in social class V as it is in social class I (Whitehead 1988). The gap in the expectation of life at birth between people in social classes I and V is about eight years, or 10 per cent of a lifetime. A recent review of poverty among children (Bradshaw 1990) found that if the average infant mortality rate had been that of social class I, 1500 fewer babies would have died in 1989, and if the UK infant mortality rate had achieved that of Sweden, 2247 fewer children would have died. Post-neonatal mortality rates in Britain are particularly high comparatively. Although infant mortality has been decreasing continuously, in recent years it has decreased more slowly in this country than among some of our neighbours – we have been overtaken. Furthermore the cause of child deaths associated with socio-economic factors has shown much less improvement, and one condition, sudden infant death syndrome, is responsible for 46 per cent of neonatal deaths. Self-reported morbidity and numerous studies based on medical observation show similar inequalities by social class (Whitehead 1988).

There is no doubt that these inequalities in health are associated with structural inequalities and with poverty that has structural origins. Factors such as poor housing, cold conditions, less safe environments, unemployment, pollution, poorer working conditions, debt, stress, poor diets and difficulties in getting access to health services are all associated with poverty and ill-health. Townsend *et al.* (1988), in a study of 678 wards in the north of England, found that 65 per cent of the variation in mortality, permanent sickness or disability, and low birth-weight could be explained by indicators of material deprivation.

Furthermore there is increasingly powerful evidence that the comparative health status of industrialized countries is not determined by the level of economic development, or by the rate of economic growth, or by the effectiveness of their health service. Nor is it the case that improvements in health can only be achieved by improvements in general living standards. The almost unanimous belief of politicians that improvements in the NHS can only be afforded out of economic growth is also wrong. In fact there is evidence (Quick and Wilkinson 1991) for arguing that it is the *distribution* of income, the *degree of inequality*, the *level of solidarity* of a nation that determines its health.

This argument is supported by evidence which shows a close correlation between income distribution and life expectancy in different countries, and the absence of a correlation between life expectancy and GNP per capita. These relationships also hold over time. Those countries who have reduced their inequalities most have shown the fastest improvements in health. Japan has become the most egalitarian country in the world and has achieved the longest life-expectancy. By contrast, the UK, which in the early 1970s was similar to Japan in income distribution and life-expectancy, has in the 1980s experienced a sharp increase in inequality and evidence of deteriorating health, including an increase in the death-rate for men and women aged 16–45. The most rapid increases in life-expectancy occurred during the World Wars. These were periods of stress and disruption but they were also periods of unprecedented solidarity, the elimination of unemployment, and a diminution in earnings differentials and differences in living standards.

Although the relationship between inequalities and health are strong, the mechanisms at work are not well understood. However, it may be that financial worries and stress, feelings of social deprivation, the undermining of confidence, diminishing self-esteem and an increasing sense of worthlessness are sharper when inequalities are pronounced, and they all affect health. Socially determined deprivation damages health. The poor who are socially isolated, lacking social support, confiding relationships and so on, are likely to be unhealthy. The conclusion is that social cohesion and a sense of solidarity are the most important determinant of health status. The best way to improve health may not be to spend more, or to spend more on health care, but rather to concentrate on redistribution or spending that reduces inequalities.

CONCLUSION

It is now the intention of policy that health and social-service authorities should purchase services on behalf of their local populations on the basis of need. In responding to that challenge the purchasers will have to determine which definition of health needs they are led by. Are they going to attempt to establish need for health, or need for health services? It appears from documentary evidence (National Health Service Management Executive 1991) that need is to be defined as 'capacity to benefit'. This implies a welcome focus on outcomes, but also suggests a rather narrow and medical vision of health investments with perhaps low priority accorded to preventive health measures and to forms of 'treatment' where the outcomes may be rather indirectly related. The emphasis is on demonstrating the efficacy – or otherwise – of current medical interventions. 'The push for change would appear to be focused on the desire to render the clinical decisions of medical experts more accountable through the test of cost effectiveness' (Lightfoot 1993).

It does not appear from the early discussion of health needs assessment or from the documents supporting the process that it will lead to a change in the attention given by the health service to distributional and equity considerations. Needs assessment has emerged from and quickly settled into the language of priority-setting, economic efficiency, cost-effectiveness and the market-orientated preoccupations of the political right.

In this chapter, I have implicitly argued that if we are to adopt a social definition of health, then we have to be engaged in research on a much wider range of issues than merely the assessment of the prevalence of medical conditions. I have presented my remarks from a social policy perspective. Social policy as a discipline or area of study has throughout its history been preoccupied with distributional issues, with the study of poverty and deprivation and the contribution of collective services and benefits to mitigating these inequities. I have not, I think, said anything which is madly original, but in contemporary debates about health care reform in Britain and elsewhere the issue of equity is too often ignored. This is well illustrated in the British government's preventive health strategy described in the document *The Health of the Nation* (Department of Health 1992). I hope that drawing attention once again to the structural causes of inequality in health will help to keep these issues on the research agenda as the research community responds to the challenge of needs assessment in the NHS.

REFERENCES

Barry, B. (1965) *Political Argument*, London: Routledge & Kegan Paul.

Black, Sir D., *et al.* (1988) *The Black Report: Inequalities in Health*, Harmondsworth: Penguin Books.

Bradshaw, J.R. (1972) 'A taxonomy of social need', in Mclachlan, G., ed., *Problems and Progress in Medical Care*, Oxford: Nuffield Provincial Hospital Trust.

—— (1990) *Child Poverty and Deprivation in the UK*, London: National Children's Bureau.

Clayton, S. (1983) 'Social need revisited', *Journal of Social Policy* 12, 2: 215–34.

Cmnd 6404 (1942) *Social Insurance and Allied Services: Report by Sir William Beveridge*, London: HMSO.

Culyer, A.J. (1992) 'Need, greed and Mark Twain's cat', in Corden, A., Robertson, G., and Tolley, K., eds, *Meeting Needs*, Aldershot: Avebury Gower.

Department of Health (1992) *The Health of the Nation*, London: HMSO.

Doyal, L., and Gough, I. (1991) *A Theory of Social Need*, London: Macmillan.

Dubos, R. (1976) 'Mirage of health: utopias, progress and biological change', in Anston, R., ed, *World Perspectives, Volume* 22, New York: Harper & Row.

Graham, H. (1987) 'Women's smoking and family health', *Social Science and Medicine* 25, 1: 47–56.

Helman, C.G. (1981) 'Diseases versus illness in general practice', *Journal of Royal College of General Practitioners* 31: 548.

Huby, M., and Dix, G. (1992) *Evaluating the Social Fund*, Social Policy Research Unit, University of York.

Ife, J. (1980) 'The determination of social need – a model of need statements in social administration', *Australian Journal of Social Issues* 15, 2: 92–107.

Illsley, R., and Le Grand, J. (1987) *Measurement and Inequality in Health*, Welfare State Programme Discussion Paper 12, London: London School of Economics.

Kaplan, C.A., and Kotler, R.L. (1985) 'Self-reports: predictive of mortality', *Journal of Chronic Diseases* 38: 195–201.

Le Grand, J. (1982) *The Strategy of Equality: Redistribution and the Social Services*, London: Allen & Unwin.

—— (1991) *The Distribution of Public Expenditure on Health Care Revisited*, Welfare State Programme Working Paper 64, London: London School of Economics.

Lightfoot, J. (1993) *Towards a Conceptual Framework of Need for Community Health Nursing: Issues of Theory and Practice in Health Needs assessment and the Setting of Priorities*, Social Policy Research Unit Paper 1071, York: Social Policy Research Unit.

Megone, C.B. (1992) 'What is need?', in Corden, A., Robertson, G., and Tolley, K., eds, *Meeting Needs*, Aldershot: Avebury Gower.

National Health Service Management Executive (1991) *Assessing Health Care Needs: A DHA Project Discussion Paper*, London: National Health Service Management Executive.

O'Donnell, O., and Propper, C. (1989) *Equity and the Distribution of National Health Services Resources*, Welfare State Programme Discussion Paper 45, London: London School of Economics.

Quick, A., and Wilkinson, R. (1991) *Income and Health*, London: Socialist Medical Association.

Robertson, P. (1991) *Rethinking Need: The Case of Criminal Justice*, Aldershot: Dartmouth.

Rowntree, B.S. (1901) *Poverty: A Study of Town Life*, London: Longmans.

Sen, A.K. (1981) *Food and Famine: An Essay on Entitlement and Deprivation*, London: Oxford University Press.

Spek, J.E. (1972) 'On the economic analysis of health and medical care in a Swedish health district', in Hauser, M., ed., *The Economics of Medical Care*, London: Allen & Unwin.

Townsend, P. (1979) *Poverty in the United Kingdom*, Harmondsworth: Penguin Books.

Townsend, P., Philimore, P., and Beattie, A. (1988) *Health and Deprivation: Inequality and the North*, London: Croom Helm.

Whitehead, M. (1988) *The Health Divide*, London: Penguin Books.

Wiggins, D. (1987) *Needs, Values and Truth*, Oxford: Blackwell.

Williams, A. (1978) 'Need – an economic exegesis', in Wright, K.G., and Culyer, A.J., eds, *Economic Aspects of Health Services*, London: Martin Robertson.

—— (1992) 'Priorities – not needs' in Corden, A., Robertson, G., and Tolley, K., eds, *Meeting Needs*, Aldershot: Avebury Gower.

World Health Organization (1985) *Targets for Health for All*, Copenhagen: World Health Organization Regional Office for Europe.

Chapter 4

Prioritizing needs with communities

Rapid Appraisal methodologies in health

Bie Nio Ong and Gerry Humphris

INTRODUCTION

The NHS reforms have redefined the role of district health authorities (DHAs) as purchasers of health care. In Chapter 1 David Hunter analyses its significance within the context of the major health service changes. In this chapter we will focus on a specific aspect of the reforms, namely the relationship between the role of DHAs (and a wider constituency of organizations contributing to the health of populations) as 'champions of the people' and the role of users of health services within the new configuration of responsibilities. If purchasers are to be the mouthpiece of the people, what strategies and methods do they employ to ensure that they are representing user views? We will analyse the concepts underlying the approach to listening to 'local voices' (National Health Service Management Executive 1992a) and outline methodologies which will enable purchasers to turn the rhetoric of championing the people's cause into reality. In doing so we will draw on a number of examples and discuss the problems associated with translating listening to people into needs profiles which can help to determine the allocation of resources.

THE POLICY FRAMEWORK

The National Health Service Management Executive (NHSME) published two documents which described the purchasers' role in needs assessment. In *Assessing Health Care Needs* health-needs assessment was seen to mean the known ability to benefit from health care, with DHAs ensuring health improvement by commissioning proven effective services (National Health Service Management Executive 1990). This disease-orientated approach was later modified by arguing that other factors were important, including epidemiological assessment, comparative assessment and a 'corporate' view taking into account the views of interested parties in order to produce an overall understanding of need (National Health Service Management Executive 1991).

Despite the recognition that health needs are not just related to health care, the dominance of the disease-based model was not fundamentally altered in other policy guidance. For example, a similar focus on the supply side can be detected in directives given to social services departments who have to formulate community care plans. They are asked to identify 'how the care needs of individuals approaching them for assistance will be assessed; how service needs identified following the introduction of systematic assessment will be incorporated into the planning process' (Department of Health 1990: 18).

The *Health of the Nation* White Paper (Department of Health 1992) and the guidance from the NHSME, *First Steps for the NHS* (1992b), broaden out from the supply-and-demand perspective into looking at health needs across health care boundaries and talk about healthy alliances with other organizations, agencies and individuals. This includes working with communities in promoting and maintaining health, targeting interventions and setting priorities.

Although national policies appear to recognize the role of users in defining health and health needs, there remains a lack of clarity about certain key concepts such as the distinction between health and health care needs (Stevens and Gabbay 1991), the relationship between health needs assessment and purchasing, the interpretation of 'local voices' and the way in which purchasers should develop working relationships with communities and users. We will focus our discussion on different purchasing models, and the way in which user involvement can be incorporated in the various approaches. A discussion of needs will not be repeated here as Jonathan Bradshaw has addressed this issue in the previous chapter.

PURCHASING MODELS AND NEEDS ASSESSMENT

The reformed National Health Service (NHS) has, in theory, given DHAs an enhanced status in that as purchasers they are able to shape health services through their purchasing action. At the same time, purchasing is a new activity, and cannot draw on established and tested approaches. Pickin and St Leger (1993) argue that health needs assessment, option assembly and option appraisal have been practised for years. Within the purchasing framework these now have to take place in a coherent manner and to be applied to the effective use of resources. They distinguish five key elements to purchasing: health-needs assessment, health resource option appraisal, prioritization, contracting, and managing the non-contract agenda.

There is little disagreement with these broad stages of purchasing, yet there is a number of interpretations of how these stages should be operationalized and how certain key dilemmas have to be resolved. To take the latter, Heginbotham and Ham (1992) outline a number of purchasing dilemmas:

1 expert vs lay opinion
2 individual need vs institutional response
3 acute vs community or primary care
4 intervention vs prevention
5 horizontal vs vertical equity
6 quality of life vs saving life
7 enhancing structural (or input) conditions vs the importance of specific health gains or outcomes.

They go on to argue that a resolution of these dilemmas would allow criteria to be defined for making allocation decisions between and within care groups by balancing a number of pressures: national policy and targets (e.g. Health of the Nation), evidence of cost-effectiveness of interventions, pressure from providers and professional groups, and public participation and local pressure.

It is important to examine how the framework for purchasing is translated into structures which allow the delivery of health care to be based on a needs assessment addressing the above dilemmas. For our discussion the specific aspects of public involvement in this process are of most importance. Difficult choices have to be made, and the public does not speak with one voice. Depending on local circumstances, balances shift, for example, from primary to acute care, from improving quality of life to saving life, and so on. One of the major difficulties in the UK is the absence of an overall decision framework which defines the central values upon which health policy is based. The example of the Dutch system, where the concept of necessary care (meaning care that makes participation in society possible) is developed, highlights explicit principles underlying choices in health care. The individual and professional approaches to health needs assessment are subordinate to the community approach. This results in a broad ethical base for decision-making, and a structured approach to public involvement in choice (Dunning 1992).

In the UK no such overarching framework guides the creation of appropriate structures for purchasing, and therefore a multitude of models has emerged. Broadly, these can be classified into joint (consortium or agency) and locality purchasing arrangements. Ham (1992) lists a number of reasons for joint purchasing, including viability, pooling skills, economies of scale, easier to form healthy alliances (that is, alliances between organizations aimed at improving health), integrated purchasing of primary, community and secondary care, and so on. In his view the obvious danger is that bigger purchasing agencies are further removed from the people they serve, and that purchasing decisions will be insensitive to local needs and will fail to take general practitioners' (GPs') views into account.

The locality purchasing model attempts to counterbalance the above drawback by combining the advantages of purchasing for a bigger population whilst remaining sensitive to the needs of small communities and client groups. Ham's research demonstrates that within the locality focus a number of approaches exists, and that locality purchasing is only one of a number of ways in which communities can be involved in purchasing decisions. The fundamental similarity lies in the commitment to develop methods for involving the broadest possible constituency in the planning, monitoring and evaluation of services. While this may include GPs, other agencies such as family health services authorities (FHSAs) – for example, the unified commissioning project described in Barking and Havering *et al.* 1992 – and social services departments, voluntary organizations and other interested parties, in the discussion we will limit ourselves to examining the role of communities within this process.

COMMUNITY INVOLVEMENT

The World Health Organization (WHO) Health for All 2000 approach has emphasized the centrality of communities in promoting their own health and in active participation in decision-making processes around priority setting and resource allocation. In terms of strategy development this implies multi-sectoral collaboration, including local communities, exemplified in the 'healthy cities' projects (Ashton 1992).

This philosophy has stimulated a renewed upsurge of community-participation projects in the health field. Many of these projects are based on the community development model, which aims to empower communities, whether they are geographical, social or cultural in nature. Generally, the work originating from this tradition uses methodologies which involve building on existing community networks and attempts to gain understanding of key local issues through working within communities. These types of methods are time-consuming and include: networking, building trust, setting agendas for action, and so on.

Two documented UK health examples are the Stockwell Health Project (Webster 1991), which was part of a larger community development programme in Lambeth between 1970 and 1984, and another London-based project using a community health survey (Dun 1990). Both projects were aimed at managers in that the results were intended to be used to aid local decision-making and inform policy-makers of local opinions. Ubido and Snee (1992) describe a variety of projects in the north-west of England employing a similar range of methods.

A number of questions can be raised in relation to these applications. They are concerned with the concept of community on the one hand, and community development methodologies on the other hand. The view of community emerging from recent government documents appears to centre around traditional relationships of family, friends and neighbours, providing people with a set of supportive relationships. Beresford and Croft (1986) offer an incisive critique of this concept of community, drawing on a large body of literature. They question the geographical dimension as the determining factor, and argue that this intersects with networks which are not spatially bounded. Feminist analysis has drawn attention to the ideological nature of the term community which renders labour within families and by women invisible, by considering it as confirmed to the private community sphere (Baldwin and Twigg 1991).

Beresford and Croft demonstrate with their research that the term 'community' conveys a sense both of space and of a focus for relationships. Interdependence within communities can be seen both as positive – that is support, cooperation, friendships – and negative – exclusion, competition, being trapped. It is important to understand the different aspects of community, and the ways in which they are perceived by particular groupings, in order to determine what local communities are and how they define their needs. Purchasers have to get sufficiently close to communities to detect the complexities and contradictions which are to inform a health-needs assessment.

Community development methodologies have a long and varied tradition, in both developed and developing countries. Although the applications have taken place in widely differing contexts, certain weaknesses in the methodologies have become apparent. First, community development is time-consuming, with relationships being forged between key people in the community and designated workers from government or other agencies. Second, the scope of community development tends to be limited in that decision-makers are not directly engaged in a dialogue with the community. Designated workers act as mediators between the community and those in power and thus can only indirectly influence policy and planning. This means that setting priorities and allocation of resources largely remain outside the domain of communities.

Purchasers who are seeking to create a locality focus and test methodologies capable of involving communities have to address the above issues. Getting close to communities is necessary in order to capture their complexity, to gain credibility and to establish a dialogue. Purchasers have to cope simultaneously with agendas which impose time constraints. Furthermore, needs assessment has to find its expression in resource allocation if purchasing is to be seen as responsive and credible. In short, involving communities means continuity – that is, establishing relationships – and action – that is, tangible outcomes.

The purchaser–provider separation has exposed the important issue of expertise in assessing needs. Professionals dominate the assessment of need of individuals and client groups as they 'ratify' expressed needs by providing a service. Furthermore, they have been able to shape needs through their own research and development actions. Now, DHAs, and public health departments in particular, have been charged with assessing the needs of populations. They draw on disciplines such as epidemiology, health economics, sociology and other social sciences, and so on, but at the same time require the clinical expertise vested in the providers.

The experience from Wales demonstrates the importance of collaboration across the purchaser–provider divide in the development of protocols which aid decision-making about priorities and resource allocation. For example, the protocol for investment in health gain in cardiovascular diseases draws on the expertise of clinicians in primary, secondary and tertiary care, voluntary and self-help groups, community health councils (CHCs), epidemiologists, health promotion experts and policy-makers (Welsh Health Planning Forum 1991). Working within such a broad constituency assists in addressing needs at the level of the individual, the client group and the population at large. Furthermore, desired action can be defined at the level of prevention and promotion, diagnosis and assessment, treatment and care, rehabilitation and health maintenance.

In summary, we argue that needs assessment requires a multidisciplinary approach which runs counter to a strict divide between purchasers and providers. The expertise held by users and communities has to be an integral part of needs assessment and to be considered alongside the public-health and clinical-needs assessments. The different inputs in the needs-assessment process offer specific and complementary insights on the complexity of needs as experienced by individuals and populations. It is within this context that we examine the contribution of methodologies which combine a community perspective and a dialogue with decision-makers on the allocation of resources.

THE RAPID APPRAISAL METHODOLOGY

In the field of rural development in Third World countries methodologies which allow for rapid, reliable and cheap profiling of community resources and characteristics have gained ground. One of the most popular methods is the Rapid Appraisal (RA), which covers many different techniques, but which has a common foundation (Conway 1988). This includes:

1 greater speed compared with conventional methods of analysis
2 working in the 'field'
3 an emphasis on learning directly from local inhabitants
4 a semi-structured, multidisciplinary approach with room for flexibility and innovation
5 an emphasis on producing timely insights, hypotheses or 'best bets' rather than final truths or fixed recommendations.

Rifkin (1992) has reviewed the application of this method within the health field, in both developing and developed countries. She discusses four major issues critical to the use of RA in the health field. First, the types of information collected in RA are predominantly qualitative in nature, and health planners used to relying on quantitative data struggle to accept its validity. This problem has been discussed within the UK context, and research design has to be opened up to accommodate the contributions based on both quantitative and qualitative perspectives (Sykes *et al.* 1992).

Second, RA has the potential to empower communities by providing new information, and also by validating information they already have. But empowerment means the ability to influence decision-making, which can result in a struggle for power and control. Planners and professionals have to recognize that ownership of the process has to be shared; and the tension between control and empowerment is, as yet, not resolved within the method (or other similar methods).

Third, information collection has to be the result of an exchange between communities and professionals, demanding a re-orientation of professional attitudes. At the same time, communities have to develop their skills and knowledge in collection and interpretation of information. This is important for the fourth aspect, namely the link between information, participation in decision-making, and establishing accountability. Rifkin argues that there is a growing tendency to connect research with decision-making which has to be based upon a strong partnership between resource holders and the designated beneficiaries.

In short, RA aims to generate information which can shape the process of resource allocation and which supports community participation. As argued previously, this approach attempts to achieve two objectives: continuity (a commitment to a community) and action (delivering tangible results).

RAPID APPRAISAL IN THE UK CONTEXT

The applications of RA within the UK have been based upon the work by Annett and Rifkin (1990). The policy framework determining its use is contextualized by the role of purchasers. The NHSME states that health authorities will have to develop the means to:

- discover and respond to the views of local people about the pattern and delivery of services – distinguishing between user view and general public opinion
- describe and explain the DHAs' objectives as they take forward service changes.

Furthermore, the tasks of FHSAs have been described in a similar way, namely as building up a unified and comprehensive picture of need (National Health Service Management Executive 1991).

As a result the RA exercises in the UK have focused on bringing the user voice into the heart of the decision-making process. Managers are required to work directly with communities in urban deprived areas (RA tends to target these because they are often least empowered). Multi-sectoral collaboration is a central tenet of the method and is based on the Health for All 2000 principles. Emphasis is placed upon understanding needs within context and in a comprehensive manner. RA offers the diverse agencies and interested parties a framework in which collaboration can take place at the level both of diagnosis and of policy-making.

RA focuses on a community's own perspective of need, which means that it uncovers the strength of feeling, rather than providing a quantitative analysis of the magnitude of a problem. The rationale is that communities will be activated when they experience a problem, and not necessarily when it has been demonstrated statistically that there is significant need. Need has to be felt by individuals or groups before it will be expressed, and thus RA has the capacity to understand both need and demand.

One of the key points for debate is how to gain access to communities and define the people who are knowledgeable about communities' problems. The RA methodology draws a purposive sample for in-depth interviews, based on the assumption that certain individuals within communities can represent different viewpoints. Their accounts of community issues reveal a number of perspectives which can be compared and contrasted in order to build up a complex and multi-layered understanding of communities. This qualitative sampling method allows in-depth analysis and can describe the form and character of needs.

The key informants to be interviewed are broadly divided into three groups:

1 people who work within a community and have a professional understanding of issues, and often interpret communities from their particular disciplinary vantage-point: for example, school teachers, police, health visitors, and so on
2 people who are recognized community leaders and seen to represent (a section of) the community: for example, councillors, church leaders, chairs of self-help groups
3 people who are important within informal networks and often play a central role in local communications: for example, a corner-shop owner, bookie, lollipop person, and so on.

It is important to realize that RA relies on other methods apart from the qualitative interview: namely, collection of secondary data (which consists of both quantitative and qualitative material), observation, geographical and social mapping, and other methods relevant within the particular exercise. Furthermore, RA in health has to be seen as part of a larger needs-assessment programme. RA focuses on subjectivity, which is limited to felt and expressed need. It cannot provide insights into the professional assessment of need; nor does it offer a comparative perspective which requires epidemiological research.

Annett and Rifkin (1990) have designed an information profile (see Figure 4.1) which systematically builds up knowledge about a community. The first level aims to gain understanding of the composition of a community, such as the demographic profile, and of how it organizes itself formally and informally in order to gauge its capacity to control

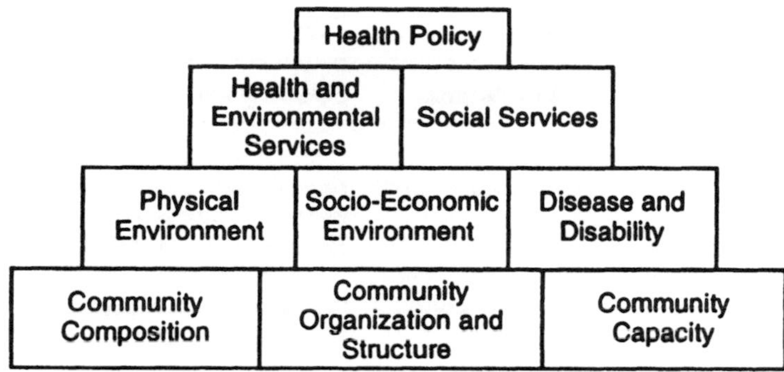

Figure 4.1 Community information profile

and maintain its own health. The second level attempts to describe the socio-ecological environment which influences health, health behaviour and the objective burden of disease and disability in a community. At the third level evidence is collated with regards to the availability, effectiveness, outcome and impact of service provision, while the final level investigates the role of policy-making in developing local strategies for health gain.

The specific tasks that have to be carried out within a RA can be schematically represented as in Table 4.1.

In summary, the UK applications of RA have followed the broad methodological outline of the original approach. The NHS reforms, and in particular the role of purchasers in assessing health needs have given RA particular poignancy in that it is a method *par excellence* for moving closer to users and communities. Specific modifications have been made in terms of sampling methods and comparing community views with those of professionals and decision-makers. Further changes will be discussed below when examining the case studies. These are in chronological order: South Sefton (Merseyside), St Helens and Knowsley, Fountain (Northern Ireland), Blythe Hill (London) and Abbey Hulton (Stoke-on-Trent).

South Sefton, Merseyside

The RA exercise in South Sefton is the first health application in a developed country and has been reported in detail elsewhere (Ong *et al.* 1991). It was part of a broader needs-assessment project which used

Table 4.1 Steps in conducting a Rapid Appraisal

Step	Task	Personnel	Comments
1	Preparation	1–2 managers	Selecting the RA team
2	2-day workshop	RA team (10–12 managers)	Choose target area Key questions identified based on information profile Respondents chosen
3	Fieldwork	3 or more small teams of researchers	Conducting interviews Preliminary analysis of data
4	1/2-day workshop	RA team	Needs list derived
5	Fieldwork	3 or more small teams of researchers	Return to respondents Priorities rank ordered by category
6	Analysis + 1/2-day workshop	RA team	Discuss results Prepare feedback meeting Formulate proposals
7	Open meeting	RA team + informants + public	Formulate concrete action plans
8	Further meeting	RA team + other managers + local community	Develop plans Evaluate actions

various other research methodologies such as a district-wide survey (Humphris *et al.* 1990), validated tools such as the Nottingham Health Profile (Hunt *et al.* 1986) and the General Health Questionnaire (Goldberg and Hillier 1979); the analysis of census and epidemiological data (Womersley and McCauley 1987); and client-group based research (Ong 1991).

The value of the RA within this context was to involve managers from a wide range of organizations – health, social services, housing – in a joint assessment and dialogue with a community that had been identified as suffering from high levels of deprivation. Against the background of the other pieces of research, the RA was able to utilize these results and place the subjective assessments of the community against the background of qualitative and quantitative findings. As such the RA did not operate within a vacuum, but could assist in focusing the planning of services on local needs, whilst not losing sight of the totality of the district population.

The lessons learned from this first RA can be summarized as follows:

- The involvement of the widest possible range of organizations should be secured in order to be able to capture and respond to the needs identified. The results demonstrated that very few needs could be identified as belonging to one agency's remit. Furthermore, a large proportion of needs were not predominantly health care needs; for example, the community's priority in the physical-environment category was the problem of rubbish.
- The emphasis in this project was on the formulation of action plans. In order to achieve this the team was made up of people who had decision-making power and tended to be rather senior within their organizations. The consequences were that these managers found it difficult to commit the time to carry out all the tasks associated with the different stages of the RA; they also tended not to be able to commit themselves in the long term (that is, beyond the formulation of action plans). Thus, while immediate change was possible through formulating and implementing specific action plans, continuing monitoring and evaluation tended to take place at a level below senior management. The community felt that the original project team did not demonstrate long-term commitment, and most of the relationships built up during the RA did not continue in existence. Credibility with the community suffered, and the RA became a tool more for diagnosis than for enduring community involvement in planning and evaluation.
- The obverse of the above, however, was that precisely because of the involvement of senior managers action plans had more chance of succeeding as each one required a shift in resources. At the same time the community had to understand the remit of the participating organizations and the constraints under which these were operating. The first three action plans formulated at the end of the RA were all completed within six months.

An important methodological change was made during this first exercise: after the fieldwork the initial formulation of a number of community

Table 4.2 Linacre ward, 1989: community priorities

	Community (N=32)	*Team professional view* (N=10)	*Team view of community* (N=10)
Physical environment			
1 Rubbish in the street	1	4	4
2 Poor quality housing	2	1	1
3 Air pollution	3	2/3	2
4 Disposal of syringes in public places	4	5	5
5 Lack of recreational space	5	2/3	3
Disease and disability			
1 Depression and anxiety	1	2	2
2 Drinking, tobacco, tranquillizers, hard drugs	2	4	3
3 Respiratory problems	3	1	1
4 Poor diet	4	3	4
Health services			
1 Lack of overall preventive children services	1	2	3
2 GPs appear 'too busy'	2	3	1
3 Lack of home support after hospital discharge	3	1	2
4 Lack of well women services	4	4	4
5 Lack of chiropody services	5	5	5
Social services			
1 Information not readily available	1	2	3
2 Lack of pre-school facilities	2	1	2
3 Fear of the power of SSDs to remove children	3	4	1
4 Home helps not free of charge	4	3	4
Socio-economic environment			
1 Unemployment	1	1	1
2 Financial problems, debt	2	3	3
3 Environment generally unsafe (e.g. robberies)	3	2	2
Community's own valuable resources			
1 Strong family support systems	1	1	1
2 Strong community action groups	2	2	3
3 'Bootle identity'	3	3	2
4 Good local councillors	4	4	4
5 Support from churches	5	5	5
6 Community Health Council	6	6	6

issues takes place. The team then returns to the people interviewed to ask them to place these issues in priority order. In the South Sefton appraisal the team members were asked to complete two priority listings before going to the community:

1 What is their own prioritization as managers or professionals?
2 What do they expect the community to prioritize (having listened to their concerns)?

These three priority lists, that is the community's, the managers and professionals' order, and their interpretation of what the community told them are shown in Table 4.2. The statistical tests used (but which are not reported here in detail) measure the level of agreement within and between groups and therefore can show the different order in priority setting. The comparison revealed that there were considerable discrepancies between professionals and community. More disturbingly, the discrepancy between the team's emphatic view of what the community told them, and the community's own perspective raised the question as to how closely the two parties can actually come together. The larger questions can be asked: to what extent can DHAs be champions of the people, and to what extent can GPs be seen as spokespeople for their patients? This debate has been touched upon by other authors, most notably Ann Bowling and colleagues (1993), who explored public and professional views in priority setting, using a survey methodology.

Thatto Heath, St Helens and Knowsley

Learning from the first exercise, the St Helens and Knowsley RA was planned using middle managers who were expected to maintain longer-term relationships with the community selected. The team was augmented by an environmental health officer, a librarian and community workers. The area chosen was Thatto Heath, being one of the most deprived estates within the district, with high unemployment and low levels of education.

The research process itself was not altered from the South Sefton one, with the exception of the priority-setting phase: the community responses were subdivided into those given by people who work but do not reside in Thatto Heath (called formal respondents) and those that live in the area (called informal respondents). The rationale for this distinction was that these two groups have different perspectives, with the former expected to express professional criteria. The team prioritized on the basis of their own professional views.

Table 4.3 Thatto Heath, 1990: community priorities

	Team	*Community*	
		Formal	*Informal*
	(N=9)	*(N=19)*	*(N=15)*
Community capacity			
Apathy	1	1	1
No community centre	2	3	2
Prejudice against 'outsiders'	4	4	4
Single parents	3	2	3
The community's own valuable resources			
Good informal information networks	2	2	2/3
Community spirit	3	3	2/3
Supportive family networks	1	1	1
Socio-economic environment			
Unemployment	1	1	1
Lack of opportunities	2	2	2
Poverty and deprivation	3	3	3
Poor education	4	4	4
Disease and disability			
Smoking and drinking	1	1	2
Acceptance of ill-health	2/3	3	3
Hard drugs	6	7	6/7
Chronic illness	7	6	4
Respiratory disease	4	2	1
Poor diet	2/3	5	5
Inadequate parenting skills	5	4	6/7
Health, social and environmental services			
Services inadequate	2	2	1
Poor information on aids/adaptions	4	4	3
No GP or chemist on the estate	3	3	4
Teenagers, nothing to do	1	1	2
Physical environment			
Pollution	6	4/5	3
Security	1	1	1
Dogs	5	4/5	7
Rats and rubbish	7	6/7	4/5/6
Dangerous roads	4	6/7	4/5/6
Inadequate housing and allocation	2	2	4/5/6
Little open space	3	3	2

The range of issues emerging in Thatto Heath were very similar to ones from Linacre ward in Liverpool. The main problem was seen to be the lack of a feeling of safety. As the data in Table 4.3 show, the three subgroups demonstrated a high level of agreement about the community's strengths and weaknesses, with a few notable exceptions. For example, the informal respondents considered pollution, inadequacy of services and chronic illness as higher priorities than both the formal respondents and the team. Opposite differences were in the following areas: inadequate housing allocation, teenagers having nothing to do, and inadequate parenting skills were considered more of a problem by formal respondents and the team than by the community.

The Thatto Heath team produced a report that was circulated to the community prior to a meeting in which a number of action plans was formulated. The report also served as a record of the problems highlighted by the exercise, and was presented to the various statutory organizations in order to assist them in longer term planning of services for the area. The problem with the latter approach was that the senior managers reading the report were not involved in the same way as the middle managers who carried out the RA. Thus, action had to be mediated through middle managers, which often meant a slow response. On the other hand, this level of management is better able to build and maintain relationships with communities and secure continuity. The inverse problem of the South Sefton experience became apparent, with a high degree of continuity through sustained relationships of trust with the community, but less capacity for action.

Fountain, Londonderry, Northern Ireland

The situation within Northern Ireland is unique within the UK in that the integrated structure of health and social care services (as organized by the Health and Social Services Boards) requires that health and social care needs are assessed together. The Western Health and Social Services Board has installed an IT computer system with trained staff as part of Northern Ireland's Needs Assessment Project (NINA). This sophisticated database of information containing health and social care activity levels will provide important epidemiological information for clinicians in public health. However, there is recognition that even sophisticated computer information systems cannot provide a full picture. The Western Health and Social Services Board from within the Foyle Community Unit has set up the Needs Assessment Research Project (NARP). The project team consists of researchers from social-work and health backgrounds and aims to provide for the unit's catchment area of 166,000 people a mechanism for acting as a bridge between professionals and ordinary people, by asking how users define need.

One of the first studies embarked upon by the NARP was the discrete housing area named the Fountain, in inner-city Londonderry. A RA method was loosely adopted; however, the team conducting the research was the professional NARP research staff, as opposed to local managers of services. The reason for this decision was the lack of time afforded to the NARP staff, as they were required to develop their procedures very quickly and to produce their first needs-assessment report for this locality. The project staff collected service provision information according to street postcodes, as well as housing and social trends from data already archived in the relevant information systems. Professional and voluntary/community groups were approached, including locality managers, GPs, health visitors, community nurses and social workers, before the Fountain residents were contacted. The participation from the local people was good.

Although the 'mini-RA' conducted in the Fountain area was not conducted with all of the recommended features of RA, the unique circumstances of the NARP within the Western Health and Social Services Board, provided some interesting lessons for the RA method. First, the benefit of having health and social services as one organization helped to prevent the conflict and bias which may distort findings within other parts of the UK that have separate health and social services components. The project staff were aware of the limitations of their original RA and decided to repeat their investigations, using a different and more intensive methodology. They employed in-depth interviews of local residents and achieved a set of results which closely conformed to their original and quick RA carried out a few months earlier.

Second, the Fountain community was able to use the 'information profile' (Figure 4.1) to identify their needs in a systematic way, as the headings for each profile block helped them to focus their attention. In the feedback to the team they highlighted that the profile was valuable in providing a framework to organize their concerns which would otherwise have been difficult to express in the brief time available in the consultation period.

Third, the representatives of the Fountain community related that they immensely enjoyed the process of outlining the planning profile. This response was likely to have led to the fourth benefit of strengthening the links between the research team and the community, thus increasing the opportunity for more intensive consultation. In conclusion, the RA provided a structured vehicle for the community to be listened to.

This assessment of the Fountain area can be considered as a partial validation of the RA technique under less than ideal procedural conditions, where researchers rather than local managers were the team of investigators.

Blythe Hill, London

All the above examples of RA have focused on a community that is predominantly geographically and culturally defined. With the emergence of GPs as an important force in the assessment of health needs other populations could be considered as vital for health profiling. There is considerable debate whether GP populations represent a coherent entity, as the only obvious unifying factor is the use of one particular primary care service. Yet, in some areas the argument could be made that GP populations are relatively coherent if they draw on communities which have very similar socio-economic backgrounds and similar disease patterns, and which are relatively compact in a spatial sense. Thus, when we were approached by an inner-city London GP practice to explore the possibility of a RA we did take it up.

The central force behind the exercise was a GP from a large group practice, and he had drawn support from the community health unit and education and social services. The RA workshop was held, using the same format as the previous workshops, and the boundaries for the community were drawn in a precise manner encompassing a community confined to the Blythe Hill area. The largest majority of GP patients were drawn from this area, and the team felt confident that the overlap between GP populations and this community was as closely matched as possible.

This RA exercise has not progressed as smoothly as the other ones because of personnel problems, and no results can be reported at this moment. We have included it within the discussion because of the change in target population, which is a departure from the previous RAs and opens up interesting discussions about the definitions of communities and the role of GPs in the assessment of need. They have to reconcile the possible contradictions within their GP catchment populations and allow for varying needs to be expressed by different communities and client groups within their overall practice population. A RA could be helpful in exploring the complexity and diversity, but the boundaries for the exercise have to be clearly defined and made explicit.

Table 4.4 Abbey Hulton, 1992: community priorities

	Team		*Community*	
	Professional	*View of community priorities*	*Formal*	*Informal*
	(N=9)	*(N=9)*	*(N=24)*	*(N=8)*
Socio-economic				
Unemployment	1	1	1	3
Poverty	2	2	2	4/5
No prospects for young people	3	3	3	4/5
Lack of parental control	4	4	4	1
Negative view of education	5	7	5	2
Teenage pregnancy	6	5	6	7
Organized bullying	7	6	7	6
Disease and disability				
Smoking	1	5	1	2
Poverty as health hazard	2	2	2	4
Young children's health	3	3	3/4	6
Asthma and respiratory disease	4	4	5	1
Alcohol	5	6	3/4	3
Drug-use	6	1	6	5
Risky sexual behaviour	7	7	7	7
Health and environmental services				
Conflicting advice between health professionals	1	4	1	2/3
Lack of facilities at health centre	2	1	2	4
Health services and staff off-putting	3	2	4	2/3
GPs not responsive	4	3	3	1
Social services				
Only available in a crisis	1/2	3	1	2/3
Lack of information	1/2	4	2/3	1
Long waiting-times for services	3	2	4	2/3
Threat of taking children away	4	1	2/3	4
Physical environment				
Feeling unsafe	1	4	1	3/4
Vandalism	2	3	2	1
Lack of policing	3	2	3	3/4
Speeding care/joy-riding	4	1	5	2
Lack of housing choice	5	5	4	5

Abbey Hulton, Stoke-on-Trent

The last example of a RA in an urban area has taken place in an inner-city area with considerable health and environmental problems. The rationale for the RA came from the health sector, which wanted to develop a programme for the prevention of heart disease. In order to target its work it was felt that a broader community profile was required of the particular population selected.

Abbey Hulton is very much like the communities from the previous RAs. One section of the patch is a designated housing-action area, where the Housing Department has carried out a lot of consultation. However, the rest of Abbey Hulton has not been subject to this exercise and therefore felt disadvantaged in that respect. This also underlined the divisions within Abbey Hulton, which could be considered as being made up of several sub-communities. The RA was aimed at understanding the common elements in the experiences of the various communities in order to arrive at a shared approach to improving the quality of life in Abbey Hulton, by offering the statutory services a handle on planning for joint action.

The team composition was the widest thus far, comprising managers from the hospital, the community and primary health care, social services, housing and education. The agenda was set as usual within a two-day workshop, and the list of priorities was derived from the field interviews with key people. A new methodological departure was that the final rankings were refined even further into:

- the perspective of the team as professionals/managers
- how the team interpreted the community perspective
- the informal respondents in the community, i.e. people who live in the community
- the formal respondents, i.e. people who work in the community.

This meant that a meta-analysis could be carried out on how the team understood the community's rankings, alongside a comparative analysis of different perspectives within the community. This multi-layered analysis, shown in Table 4.4, allowed for a detailed discussion with the community on the various interpretations, and highlighted both the differences and the similarities in the community. The issues that emerged appeared very much like the ones from the Linacre and Thatto Heath exercises. The pattern, however, showed some differences:

The results can be broken down in three ways:

1 inspecting the priorities themselves as listed under each category of

the planning profile. Essentially the priorities which ensue from the RA process may be considered to be the most valuable data;

2 examining the level of agreement by Kendall's Coefficient of Concordance within each of the sets of 'judges' when they were invited to rank order the priorities in each of the categories
3 comparing the ranks across the set of 'judges' for each priority listed.

The priorities that were identified from the interviews conducted with the community informants showed that many of the areas that were identified in previous RAs were found to be present in the Abbey Hulton RA. For instance, the priorities of unemployment, drug abuse, respiratory diseases and lack of safety within the local area are parallel concerns in virtually all RAs reported to date. Some priorities, however, focused upon by this community were unique, and probably reflected an aspect of the time in which the RA was conducted. A good example, which appeared to reflect media attention as well as the concerns of the community studied, was the problem of 'joy-riding' and the resulting health hazards.

The levels of agreement for the staff's rank ordering of their own priorities for Abbey Hulton was poor, with only the socio-economic category showing significant agreement among the staff group. By comparison, the community participants scored higher on agreement, with many of the categories demonstrating a significant level of concordance, especially with the formal informants. This set of results tends to parallel the previous RAs in Linacre and Thatto Heath.

Of interest are the differences between the team's expectations of the community priority ranking and their own view of how priorities should be ranked. In addition, direct comparisons can be made with the community's views. The most statistically significant comparison was the 'negative view of education' category, which referred to the poor perception of current educational standards and opportunities offered by the local educational services. The team and the community differed: the team believed that the community would rank educational priority comparatively low; the perception of the community, and especially the 'informal' members, appeared to contradict the team's belief, as they ranked education appreciably higher than what the team expected. The difference between the team and community views may be explained by the focus of the media on the National Curriculum at the time of the RA, which could have heightened concern among Abbey Hulton residents. Such an effect would confirm one of the original premises of RA, in that the method provides a 'snapshot' of a community's assessment of their needs, rather than a stable set of priorities unaffected by temporary changes. It also raises the issue of the cyclical nature of needs assessment, which requires regular evaluation against actions, achieved goals and evolving perceptions of populations.

A further example of the disparity between the team's understanding of the community's priorities and the community's own ranking appeared in the social services category. The team believed that a major issue for residents was the perceived threat of the power of social services to remove children from 'unsuitable' families. The informal community participants rated this issue the least important problem associated with social services.

Our final example demonstrated some consistency with other RAs in relation to the use of drugs. In Abbey Hulton, similarly to Thatto Heath, smoking and alcohol were introduced as separate items. However, in Abbey Hulton illicit drug-use was included as a priority under the heading of 'Disease and disability'. In common with previous RAs, the team rated drug-use as a community concern, while both sets of community respondents rated the issue fairly low on their list of items

The Abbey Hulton exercise was systematic in preparation and execution. The experience from previous RAs helped in the decision-making process, for instance, in the selection of team members and community respondents. Among the most important alterations was the recommendation to collect data from the team, and splitting the informants into two groups – informal and formal. Subsequent analysis showed precise distinctions which confirmed similarities with previous RAs, demonstrating the generalizability of health needs in deprived areas, alongside distinct and specific concerns pertaining to Abbey Hulton.

CONCLUSION

Assessing the needs of populations is a complex endeavour. Purchasers have to develop methods alongside the traditional existing approaches of public health departments if they are to understand the totality of need. Moreover, as they are compelled by government guidance to involve users in this process they have to respond with creative methods to make this possible.

In this chapter, we have addressed two issues: one regarding method, and another regarding execution. To take the latter first, there is considerable uncertainty as to the present capacity of public health departments to undertake the task set for them in needs assessment, and especially as to whether they are capable of understanding unmet need and demand, the cultural diversity of need and the possible contradictions between needs expressed by different groupings (or individuals). The danger with the emergence of larger purchasing consortia is that, instead of moving closer to the user, the opposite happens and purchasers are becoming further removed.

The role of the providers in assessing needs remains important: not only do they have direct contact with users; they also have accumulated knowledge about service uptake, the context in which service delivery takes place and the effectiveness of certain interventions. Within the strategic framework of *The Health of the Nation* (Department of Health 1992) purchasers and providers have to exploit this expertise and jointly design needs assessment methodologies.

Concerning method, the rhetoric of user involvement requires a fundamental rethinking of the relationship between decision-makers and users. It is not sufficient to see users as consumers who are satisfied or dissatisfied with services. The place of the users is in the joint definition of need, priority setting, and evaluation. This approach means a paradigm shift whereby the community perspective will be used as the guiding principle for setting priorities in health care and a broad social consensus should be achieved (Dunning 1992). The RA attempts to do this on a small scale, but there is scope to extrapolate to larger entities, depending on the strategic choice of opting for a community perspective of need. Consequently, methods will become collaborative efforts between a range of managers and users (in the widest sense, including potential users, carers and social networks). Following the involvement of users in diagnosis and planning, action and continuing evaluation are the necessary tangible outcomes of this joint working if it is to survive beyond a short project life. The RA method has the potential for being developed into a tool that involves communities directly and fundamentally in defining health needs and health gains, and thus in the process of decision-making.

REFERENCES

Annett, H., and Rifkin, S. (1990) *Improving Urban Health*, Geneva: World Health Organization.

Ashton, J., ed. (1992) *Healthy Cities*, Milton Keynes: Open University Press.

Baldwin, S., and Twigg, J. (1991) 'Women and community care – reflections on a debate', in Maclean, M., and Groves, D., eds, *Women's Issues in Social Policy*, London: Routledge.

Barking and Havering FHSA and Barking, Havering and Brentwood Health

Authority (1992) *Commissioning of Primary and Community Health Services 1992*, Essex: Unified Commissioning Project.
Beresford, P., and Croft, S. (1986) *Whose Welfare?* Brighton: The Lewis Cohen Urban Studies Centre.
Bowling, A., Jacobson, B., and Southgate, L. (1993) 'Health service priorities: Explorations in consultation of the public and health professionals on priority setting in an inner London health district', *Social Science and Medicine* 37, 7: 851–7.
Conway, G. (1988) 'Editorial', *Rapid Rural Appraisal Notes* 1: 2.
Department of Health (1990) *Community Care in the Next Decade and Beyond. Policy Guidance*, London: HMSO.
—— (1992) *The Health of the Nation*, London: HMSO.
Dun, R. (1990) 'What the people say', *Health Service Journal*, 5 April: 518–19.
Dunning, A. (1992) *Choices in Health Care*, Rijswijk: Ministry of Welfare, Health and Cultural Affairs.
Goldberg, D., and Hillier, V. (1979) 'A scaled version of the General Health Questionnaire', *Psychological Medicine*, 9: 139–45.
Ham, C. (1992) *Locality Purchasing*, Birmingham: Health Services Management Centre.
Heginbotham, C., and Ham, C. (1992) *Purchasing Dilemmas*, London: King's Fund College.
Humphris, G., Ong, B.N., and others (1990) *Health and Lifestyle: A Survey in South Sefton*, Liverpool: Priority and Community Care Unit.
Hunt, S., McEwen, P., and McKenna, S. (1986) *Measuring Health Status*, London: Croom Helm.
National Health Service Management Executive (1990) 'Assessing health care needs', DHA Project Paper, June, London.
—— (1991) 'Moving forwards – needs, services and contracts', DHA Project Paper, March, London.
—— (1992a) 'Local voices: the views of local people in purchasing for health', January, London.
—— (1992b) *First Steps for the NHS*, London: National Health Service Management Executive.
Ong, B.N. (1991) 'Researching needs in district nursing', *Journal of Advanced Nursing* 16: 638–47.
Ong, B.N., Humphris, G., Annett, H., and Rifkin, S. (1991) 'Rapid Appraisal in an urban setting: an example from the developed world', *Social Science and Medicine* 32, 8: 909–15.
Pickin, C., and St Leger, S. (1993) *Assessing Health Need Using the Life Cycle Framework*, Buckingham: Open University Press.
Rifkin, S. (1992) 'Rapid Appraisal for health', *Rapid Rural Appraisal Notes*, July: 7–12.
Stevens, A., and Gabbay, J. (1991) 'Needs assessment needs assessment', *Health Trends* 23, 1: 20–3.
Sykes, W., Collins, M., Hunter, D., Popay, J., and Williams, G. (1992) *Listening to Local Voices*, Leeds: Nuffield Institute for Health; Salford: Public Health Research and Resource Centre.
Ubido, J., and Snee, K. (1992) *Consumer Participation Directory of Projects*,

Merseyside and Chester, Observatory Report Series, 12, University of Liverpool.
Webster, G. (1991) 'Community development and health: a collective approach to social change', paper presented at the BSA Annual Conference, March, Manchester.
Welsh Health Planning Forum (1991) *Protocol for Investment in Health Gain: Cardiovascular Diseases*, Cardiff: Welsh Office.
Womersley, J., and McCauley, D. (1987) 'Tailoring health services to the needs of individual communities, *Journal of Epidemiology and Community Health* 41: 190–5.

Part III

Public involvement in research on health

Chapter 5

The power of lay knowledge

A personal view

Meg Stacey

INTRODUCTION

All of us are perhaps most familiar with the power of lay knowledge in the negative sense of stopping things happening – or at least trying to. This is often what professionals, particularly doctors and nurses, notice most. It is what they refer to as non-compliance. People who fail to turn up for outpatients, people who fail to bring their children to the child health clinic, people who do not complete the course of pills as prescribed – people who refuse to conform in a variety of ways. We know that very often such people have good reasons. Not taking your child to the cold and draughty child health clinic on a pouring wet day is health-giving rather than health-denying. That's part of the intelligent use of lay knowledge.

There are also protests: protests like those of women against their treatment in childbirth, which began in that period when government, at the behest of the Royal College of Obstetricians and Gynaecologists (Department of Health and Social Security 1970), was encouraging all of us to have our babies in hospital and when the obstetricians were introducing the active management of labour. There was a great uprising about that. Then there are the many struggles against hospital closures which tend to be written off as 'those stupid local people defending that little community hospital' and seen as a kind of nuisance. (Ironically, in the new National Health Service (NHS) such hospitals are again becoming respectable.) I have also noticed that where the protest movement on behalf of local people is about a major teaching hospital they are not written off in quite the same way. Part of the trouble here is that protests about closures seem conservative to those who are planning change. They assert their own knowledge, labelling the protests as sentimental and a product of the small minds of people who can't see beyond their locality. Other protesters want change, but in ways which are offensive or disruptive to professionals or planners; although such protests may sometimes in the end make those people bend or mend their ways.

To illustrate how things have changed and to begin to indicate how we have reached our present dilemmas, let me illustrate by using some examples of lay health care action which I have been involved in during my life, a period spanning something like thirty-five years, I suppose. I think of the care-of-children-in-hospital movement in which I was involved in Swansea around 1959 as a young mother. We were trying to do that apparently very simple thing of having the hospital doors open to allow us to be with our children for more than a few hours or half-hours a week. Or even perhaps only to be able to see them by peering through the windows of an infectious diseases hospital. At that time such ideas were thought of as quite new and cheeky – challenging the received wisdom, knowledge and practice of the hospital and its staff.

How much that contrasts with the situation now, when the views of the so-called consumer are supposed to be taken into account in health-care planning and delivery. Such consultation is also very different from our experience when we went to the Hospital Management Committee asking the members if they would humanize the care of children in hospital (Platt Report 1959). We went in a spirit of cooperation to make suggestions. We were not being antipathetic. Ultimately we met the chair(man) of the management committee, who said 'What are your complaints?', and we said, 'We don't have complaints, we want to make suggestions. We think it would be better for the children if . . . '. 'But what is your complaint?' There was no place for lay suggestions in the NHS at that time and in that place. So we had to learn to couch our case in their terms. That is to say, we had to bring forward individual cases of where we thought a child or her mother had been treated inappropriately and make complaints case by case: date, time, ward, hospital staff involved. We were forced into their mould, which had no place for people who were neither professionals nor administrators but who, out of their lay knowledge and experience, were wanting to make suggestions for the improvement of the hospital.

So that particular group in South Wales insisted on working entirely cooperatively, not to say deferentially, with administrators, managers and doctors. Progress was very slow. Nationwide the big changes which finally took place were perhaps influenced by the two pieces of research that we did from Swansea University College about the care of children in hospital, but were influenced strongly by the work of James Robertson and the Save the Children Fund, which put its weight behind humanizing hospital care. Years later I said that if we had that time over again I would have recommended direct action in order to make people understand just how seriously we felt – like sitting on the management committee's doorstep, or some other visible demonstration. But that was not the way people worked at all in those days. It was not part of the ethos in 1960; 1968 was yet to come. There was little space for radical change in the health care system then. It has perhaps had too much radical change since (but that is another story).

So now, in 1993, there have been many changes, and everyone in the whole health care system is charged with a responsibility to listen to the consumer voice and the local voice. Some similarities remain. This new responsibility has been put upon all in the health service by government fiat, just as were the instructions to let mothers into the ward. The staff in the children's wards didn't understand why, as they saw it, they suddenly had to have their whole wards invaded by 'visitors', and their routines disrupted by these dreadful messy, untidy mothers coming in. Furthermore, they were not given the tools to do the job, so to say – no training or preparation, no physical space or equipment provided. It was very hard for them. So now we are told to involve the consumer: clearly there are all sorts of problems for health care personnel in that, and some in-built contradictions. The need to understand what the change is about is obviously still there, because there can be a lot of problems in working with local people or lay people.

In what follows in this chapter I propose to address three themes: the nature of knowledge, people's and professionals'; relationships between different kinds of knowledge; and power and knowledge in people–professional relationships. In conclusion I shall try and take a forward look at how NHS authorities and health workers may begin to grapple with these difficult issues. Before I proceed, however, I need to spell out two assumptions that will underlie what I have to say.

ASSUMPTIONS

Equality of worth

My first assumption is that all people are of equal worth whatever may be any appearances to the contrary and/or prejudices that we hold about each other. Many times in the past I have heard in a child health clinic that dismissive 'What else can you expect from a social class V mum?'

from paediatrician or clinical medical officers. In this way the professional immediately writes off such a mother as of low worth, some sort of hopeless working-class woman, one who can be expected to act unreasonably and irresponsibly. Any need to examine what might lie behind the offending behaviour is automatically excluded by the prejudiced assumption. My assumption is that any one woman is as worthy as any other, whatever categorization she may be given on the basis of her husband's occupation. Her views are as worthy of being listened to with respect as those of anyone else.

This is a political, moral and also spiritual assumption, not perhaps provable by the canons of positivist science, but one which I would argue strongly is the basis which makes it possible for people to build a decent life together and which is necessary for a decent health care system. The assumption is, after all, one which is also expressed in the long-standing British tradition of equality before the law. The principle of equality before the law, although it may be transgressed, can be claimed and re-claimed. Such a principle in terms of equal access to health care when it is needed was after all a crucial part of the very basis on which the NHS was first set up – a collective responsibility to see that the sick and suffering received treatment whatever their social situation might be.

People as health producers

My second assumption is of a different order and has to do with the nature of health work: it is that people – the public, patients and potential patients – are as much producers as they are consumers of health care. Much is said nowadays about consumers: people do 'consume' health care, but they also produce health and health care. I have for many years argued that in the health care system the consumer and the producer are one (Stacey 1976, 1981, 1984, 1988). A doctor cannot treat patients without their input; the role of each in the health production process may be different, but both are crucial. Indeed, in all service industries the client is a producer as well as a consumer.

What is drummed into us is our responsibility for our own health – to brush our teeth and not smoke and to control our alcohol intake – but 'patients as producers' goes beyond that. Patients do a great deal of hard work. This is very obvious in the case of labouring mothers producing babies. High-tech medicine has created even more work for patients to do, maintaining the apparatus attached to them (as in stoma care, for example), or to which they are attached (as in the case of home renal dialysis) (Strauss *et al.* 1982). Technology creates a particular kind of patient work, but patients always have to work. Doctors and nurses have known for many years that a patient who does not wish to live will die in the end despite their best efforts, although oddly enough that may come about more slowly now with modern technological medicines than it did before.

We are also producers of each other's health as well as our own; we are all (unpaid) health workers. Women in particular are responsible for the health of their families. This comes out clearly in the recently published account of two local women's protest movements: a group of housing tenants and a group of miners' wives studied in Bradford by Susan Hyatt (1992). She calls her book *Putting Bread on the Table*. The title comes from the account that Jean, one of her respondents, was telling her about how she became involved in the miners' wives' movement during that great strike in 1984/5. The men said to Jean, 'Our lasses are not interested in politics', to which she replied, 'I am not talking about politics, I am talking about putting bread on the table', which was the real problem that women had in the strike (Hyatt 1992: 7). And, as Hyatt indicates, the responsibility of women for putting bread on the table goes to the heart of women's politics. It also goes to the heart of women's concerns about health: their health, their children's health and their partners' health. This is because, traditionally, it has been the prime responsibility of women to keep their family healthy and treat those who fall sick. So women *par excellence* are health care producers; they are unpaid health workers, and we should think of them in that way. And so are the very many men who take care not only of themselves in maintaining their own health, but also of aged parents or sick wives, and the increasing, but still too small, number who share with women the health promoting activities of the home.

The crucial point which flows from this understanding is that unpaid health workers are part of the health team. Historically, however, they have been treated as 'the other', the people out there, the people that can create a nuisance when they don't conform, when they don't comply with the latest professional ideas.

KEY THEMES

Professional knowledge and people knowledge

On the whole I prefer to speak of 'people knowledge' rather than 'lay knowledge'. This is because 'lay' (even though it originally comes from a Greek word meaning 'of the people') tends to be what is used for those people who do not belong to a specific profession, particularly those who are not clerics and medics. In referring to people who lack particular qualifications or have not been ordained, 'lay' suggests the absence of something valuable or prestigious, and may imply less competence, or even less moral worth. Thus it underlines the very distinction I wish to argue is false except in a limited technical sense.

The main distinction between professional and people knowledge is that the latter is most often experiential knowledge. It derives from what people experience. This knowledge is not necessarily either simple or *simplest*; it may be quite complex, as Hyatt's research indicates. However, people knowledge is not that sort of knowledge which is codified in books or taught in university lecture theatres or in schools; it is not systematized and generalized as professional knowledge is. Those beliefs and understandings about health and illness, the essence of people's experiences, are modified and passed on, mostly by word of mouth, and offend against positivistic canons by including the subjective along with the objective. In health care matters, people knowledge includes a good deal of medical knowledge which has been acquired as a part of experience. Sometimes people knowledge derives from that of an earlier period of medical knowledge, intermixed with experience of more recent medical practice. But its crucial characteristics are that it is informal, experiential and mostly unwritten.

Relationships between different kinds of knowledge

I remember arguing with a research body, a steering committee overseeing some research about childbirth. It was trying to find out whether, if a pregnant woman were asked to count and record the times she felt her baby kick in the womb, the data would provide an early warning of the possible death of the baby *in utero*. The plan involved a counting timetable and a hotline to the hospital if the kicks went below a specified number. I suggested the researchers might also open the hot-line to women who just wanted to say, 'I think the baby isn't right', or 'I haven't felt it', or something similar – not only when the kicks as counted conformed to the doctors' criteria. But, no, that was not allowed. The expert medical advisers seemed to feel that if one opened the line in that way all the pregnant women in the sample would be bombarding the hotline.

This people–professional difference seemed to have a number of aspects. There was a presumption that the women lacked the ability to distinguish between transitory and more profound changes, and also presumed a high level of 'neuroticism' among the women. There is a connection too with the way in which obstetricians have changed how our babies are perceived in the womb. We used to understand by feel, but the obstetricians, not having our experience of feelings, were constrained to look, first peering in, then using X-rays and later ultrasound. So now we women have to see too, but we see through other people's eyes on the ultrasound. What the doctors see in this view is the foetus *in utero*, part of the interior of a woman – the rest of her disappears from view.

People have experiential knowledge about bad or polluted environments which is different from the scientists' knowledge; scientific measurements may not reveal correlations that people believe exist between respiratory diseases, for example, and the pollutants in the environment or the dampness in the houses. My favourite story along those lines comes from the Lower Swansea Valley project (Hilton 1967). The epidemiological team spent a lot of time trying to measure the pollution in the lower valley, the inefficiency of housing, and what the connections were with ill-health. They failed to come up with any meaningful correlations, but in the process one of the team developed chronic bronchitis which proved extremely intractable.

Power and knowledge in people–professional relations

This problem about what counts as evidence can lead to other problems in the relationship between the people and the professional. I mentioned earlier how in those first protests about the treatment of children in hospital we had to behave in the way the management committee wanted us to – our suggestions had to become complaints. Our collective concern as parents, mostly mothers but also one or two fathers, had to be expressed as individual complaints about staff, action X on day Y, or problems experienced by particular parents. Because of this pressure to put lay understanding and lay experience into official language or to use acceptable research methods, various local and national groups and protest movements sometimes invite trained researchers on to their side. Sometimes trained community workers may be put in to help strengthen or improve localities. A variety of relationships may result, which need to be understood.

These have only become clearer to me over time and with experience. The trained researcher or worker may be the servant of the group, offering technical advice but accepting the group's leadership. Whether the researcher has such a technical advisory role depends on the strength of the group and how deferential or assertive it is. Another possibility is that the group may be coopted or incorporated into the goals of the professionals. A third possibility is that apparently independent groups may be engineered by professionals. Doctors wishing for greater resources for their specialty have been known to create a group of supportive patients or their relatives or to coopt an existing protest group. The risk the professional takes here is that the group may later take on a life of its own, possibly to the embarrassment of the people who engineered it.

The first time that I actually worked with local people doing research was in the Workers' Educational Association (WEA) in Banbury back in 1948. This was nothing to do with health; we were doing a social survey of the town. It began with the WEA class collecting data about their own place and expressing their views, but in the end my colleagues and I took over as professionals and did a more sophisticated study. It partly lost its contact with the direct local voices because we mediated them as researchers.

In the end I got very guilty about Banbury, which I studied twice. I found when we went back the second time that, partly because there was this base data (extremely rare in the 1950s) which my colleagues and I had collected, and also because of the proximity of Banbury to places like London, Birmingham and Oxford where researchers hailed from, the area had been re-researched and over-researched. Anybody wanting to do market research, or to do research for which they needed general social background data, dumped it there. I felt rather bad that I had started that off (*Tradition and Change: A Study of Banbury* (1960) was, after all, the book that made my academic reputation). The refusal to cooperate with surveys increased. I fully understood that protest; people were being exploited – and not in their own interest, but for the market interest of some company or other, as well as by well-meaning planners and similar policy-makers.

In the case of the protest about children in hospital I belonged to the Association for the Welfare of Children in Hospital – which was the name our Welsh group had long before the National Association for the Welfare of Children in Hospital (NAWCH) changed theirs from Mother Care for Children in Hospital (MCCH). I was a member, but also a sociologist who saw the need for sociological research – the research on which the government policy was based was entirely psychological. In planning the change the then Ministry of Health had not taken social factors about letting mothers into hospital into account at all: none of the social implications for the mothers of having to go to hospital with their sick child and leave others at home. This lack of social understanding and of staff preparation explained the refusal of nurses and doctors to accept the unrestricted presence of mothers.

I was uneasy about being involved in a political movement and researching it at the same time. There were all the problems of objectivity or detachment on the one hand and involvement and commitment on the other. There was also the question of what others might think, whether they would feel the research was biased from the outset and decry it. There was a sense, too, in which that study did objectify the respondents, and I think its approach would be outlawed by some contemporary sociologists (Prout 1979). We looked at the children rather than ask them questions, though some of them were much too small to talk to. The inspiration of the research, even if the methods were not quite consistent with it, was the experience of the children and the mothers – but we were, if you like, looking at their experiences rather than learning directly from their experiential knowledge (Stacey *et al.* 1970; Hall and Stacey 1979).

To come up to date, a quite different relationship is one that I had and still have with the Bristol Survey Support Group. This illustrates rather different points about people knowledge and people power, and relationships with official knowledge. Readers may remember some adverse research about the Bristol Cancer Help Centre published in the *Lancet* by Bagenal *et al.* (1990). The research indicated that women with breast cancer who went to Bristol were more likely to relapse and more likely to die – rather horrible and startling figures. A group of us got together at a medical sociology conference and concluded this was bad research from a professional point of view; our professional knowledge taught us that. The researchers had no grounds for coming to the conclusions they published. We also thought the way the research findings had been broadcast on television and radio and published in the press was extraordinarily inhumane. As a result of that meeting a letter objecting to the research on scientific grounds was sent to the press with fifty-five social science signatories from our group.

The really important thing, however, was the action, based on the experiential knowledge of some of the women who had been sampled in the research. A number of these breast-cancer survivors were so upset at the slur to the Bristol Centre, which they felt had helped them immensely, and also so offended about being treated as digits, about having their possible future just blazoned over the radio and the television without even being told, that they formed a protest group aimed at having the research stopped, the results totally withdrawn and an apology given. They were, I think, what Hyatt calls 'accidental activists' (Hyatt 1992: 4). The women were turned into activists because of their experience.

In this conflict there are two sets of knowledge problems: one about different types of healing knowledge; the other between women and professionals. Orthodox biomedical understanding of cancer and its treatment, including the goals of treatment, is at odds with that of the complementary therapists and spiritual healers who were working at the Bristol Cancer Help Centre. Orthodox medicine and its researchers have a heavy investment in existing practice and procedure. As soon as the women read the results they said: 'This simply cannot be true – we know it is not true.' They themselves had knowledge and experience. They knew that some of their women friends who had also been to Bristol had died. They knew that no 100 per cent cure was on offer. They hoped and worked for cure for themselves but that was not what they had been led to expect. They knew, however, that Bristol had helped them because it had empowered them. As they said when we asked the group how they had done all this: 'We were empowered.' They could not believe research which claimed Bristol had harmed them: it did not fit in with their own knowledge and experience.

As to the second knowledge question, the relation between the women and the professionals, the statisticians and others doing the study had used the sample women from the Centre extraordinarily badly. They had treated them simply as objects and had forgotten any civilized ethical code. The women, incidentally, are the first group of patients to get together and complain about their treatment as research objects. That is a very important development. So, far from being digits or objects, the women have done incredible things: they did their own research; they uncovered some dubious actions being taken; they made officials open doors and give them data. When you say to them 'Well, where have you got the strength from to do all this?', they say again: 'It is what we learned in Bristol, they gave us power.' When thinking about empowerment it is important to take note of what one of Hyatt's respondents said: 'You can't give people power, they have to take it' (Hyatt 1992: 21). That's what the Bristol women did. They took it.

Nevertheless, despite all they had done, that group who joined together as the Bristol Survey Support Group (BSSG) turned to us as medical social scientists to help them. They came to us to ask for our help and support because we had made a protest about the research being inappropriate, a public protest. In the face of everything that the women had done that made me feel extremely humble. I did not really think that there was anything very much that we could offer, and I felt they did not really need us. However, there was technical help that we could give and we were willing to give that when asked. I could also see to my regret that in an elitist society, if they had a professor, even a female one, prepared to stand up in public and say 'That research was bad, it was inappropriate, and it was unethical to treat women like that', some prestige might be added to their cause.

It is inevitable that there will from time to time be conflict between people and professionals: their perceptions and interests will not always run together. We should, however, not make the mistake of imagining that all professionals involved in any particular situation will necessarily agree among themselves, nor all of the people either. There can be inter- and intra-professional conflict deriving from different knowledge, experience and interests; members of the public will also differ as to their understanding of a problem. However, when people use their knowledge to say 'The way things are is wrong, we want them changed, or we want an apology for those actions', it is not comfortable for the professionals, and they find it difficult to perceive that the information and opinions are valuable data to be assimilated for the better running of the service.

CONCLUSION

In conclusion I shall try and draw out some lessons from this discussion of people knowledge which may be helpful for health service workers charged with the responsibility to take the 'consumer' view into account. Doubtless health workers in the thick of it will be much better able to do that for themselves than I am, but the following thoughts may start the process.

The first and most important point is that at all times one should have respect for people knowledge – for lay knowledge. A first reaction may understandably be 'They don't understand' and a feeling of helplessness that meaningful communication may never be achieved. But just stop and think 'Could it be that I don't understand their knowledge-base?' The aim should be to understand the people's point of view in their terms (not yours) and to work out where they are coming from. Only then will you be able to convey your own view of the situation in ways salient to them; or, alternatively, you may realize it needs rethinking. After all, as Robert Merton said years ago, those of us who have undergone long and thorough education have as a consequence a 'trained incapacity' (Merton 1957: 198). It can also be helpful to remember that while each health worker may be an expert in their own area, faced with expertise of another kind they are just one of the people. The division between people and professional is not a rigid one. Each one of us is sometimes people and sometimes professional.

For all of us it is also important to recall the major ideological justification for professionalism, namely service. High training is not a qualification for arrogance, although characteristics of our elitist society pull us in that direction. The best way we can each think of ourselves – and in all this I include myself, doctors, managers and all health service staff – is as technicians highly trained in one aspect of health care whose job it is to provide a service to other people. But those other people are also making their input into the health-giving process. Part of our job is to work with them to maximize that input.

An ironic aspect of the newly rearranged health service is that, despite all the rhetoric about the 'consumer' and patients' and citizens' charters, the patients, potential patients and people are further away than ever from the management and organization of the service. There seems to be an inherent contradiction between the managerial structures and the consumer rhetoric. This of itself will inevitably make for difficulties, as has already happened in the so-called 'gagging clauses' which make it dangerous for health service employees to speak out when they see things are going wrong.

Given the way managerialism is working out, a very great deal is going to depend on personnel at unit level who come into contact with patients and public in the course of arranging and providing services. In terms of formal consultation it seems unlikely that one can expect a high response. The other day I heard the chair of a community health council complaining loudly because there had only been one member of the public present at a meeting about setting up a Trust. People knowledge has taught the public in that area that at the present time, whether they went to meetings or not, the trust-making process would inexorably continue for the time being, having been ordained by a higher power. In other words, they are alienated. The political decisions are already made, and people's reaction to them makes meaningful consultation difficult if not impossible at that level. Where it is possible is where people have concerns about the provision of a service or its non-provision. Many small-scale interactions about specific issues conducted in an open spirit would seem to be the way forward.

A quite difficult problem in assessing the appropriate health provision for a locality is going to be the possibility of inadequacies hidden in people's homes. This came to me forcibly when I recently visited an excellent hospital for elderly patients, used largely as a staging-post after an illness episode and before return to their own homes or to other suitable accommodation. The contrast with those geriatric hospitals I used to visit when I first started doing work in health care was great; I rejoiced at the much greater humanity and sophistication of the care. However, as I went home I reflected on how during my life I have too often noticed that when one social problem has been removed it has tended to be transferred elsewhere away from its original locale or to reappear in a different form. Slum clearance is the most obvious example which came to mind. Fears about an inadequately funded community care service filled my mind, and the possibility of poor care or neglect hidden in myriad homes frightened me. The danger of 'out of sight out of mind' could be as great as, if not greater than, it was in the days of the great shut-away.

Not to want to know is an understandable tendency amid all the difficulties and changes of the present period. After all, there will surely be more than enough work to do without looking too closely. However, disasters lie in that direction. People power helped by professional authority may well be needed to forestall them, because what the unpaid health workers have to say will be of crucial importance if awareness is to be maintained. The dynamic which government has released in consumer consultation may be sensitively used in this context.

In making their recommendations about consumers, I am not sure that government understood that consumers are also producers, and that people knowledge is a consistent kind of rational knowledge. The people in between, the coalface workers and the unit managers, may well find themselves faced with difficulties. However, a good understanding of how and why the problems arise may be helpful in sustaining the ethic of professional *service* and ensuring enhanced health care delivery. However events unfold, in encouraging the consumer voice government politicians may find that they have got more than they bargained for.

REFERENCES

Bagenal, F.S., Easton, D.F., Harris, E., Chilvers, C.E.D., and McElwain, T.J. (1990) 'Survival of patients with breast cancer attending Bristol Cancer Help Centre', *The Lancet* 336: 606–10.

Department of Health and Social Security (1970) *Domiciliary Midwifery and Maternity Bed Needs: Report of the Sub-Committee* (Peel Report), Standing Maternity and Midwifery Advisory Committee, London: HMSO.

Hall, D., and Stacey, M., eds (1979) *Beyond Separation: Further Studies of Children in Hospital*, London: Routledge & Kegan Paul.

Hilton, K.J., ed. (1967) *The Lower Swansea Valley Project*, London: Longman Green.

Hyatt, S.B. (1992) *'Putting Bread on the Table': The Women's Work of Community Activism*, Occasional Paper no 6, Work and Gender Research Unit, Department of Economic and Social Studies, Bradford: University of Bradford.

Merton, R.K. (1957) *Social Theory and Social Structure*, London: Collier, Macmillan (Free Press of Glencoe).

Platt Report (1959) *Welfare of Children in Hospital*, London: HMSO.

Prout, A. (1979) 'Children and childhood in the sociology of medicine', paper given to the BSA Medical Sociology Conference, University of Warwick (mimeo).

Stacey, M. (1960) *Tradition and Change: A Study of Banbury*, London: Oxford University Press.

—— (1976) 'The health service consumer: a sociological misconception?', in Stacey, M., ed., *Sociology of the National Health Service*, Sociological Review Monograph no. 22, Keele: University of Keele.

—— (1981) 'The division of labour revisited or overcoming the two Adams', in Abrams, P., Deem, R., Finch. J., and Rock, P. eds, *Practice and Progress: British Sociology 1950–1980*, London: Allen & Unwin.

—— (1984) 'Who are the health workers? Patients and other unpaid workers in health care', *Economic and Industrial Democracy* 5: 157–84. London: Sage.

—— (1988) *The Sociology of Health and Healing: A Textbook*, London: Unwin Hyman.

Stacey, M., Dearden, R., Pill, R., and Robinson, D., eds (1970) *Hospitals, Children and their Families: The Report of a Pilot Study*, London: Routledge & Kegan Paul.

Strauss, A.L., Fagerhaugh, S., Suczec, B., and Weiner, C. (1982) 'The work of hospitalized patients', *Social Science and Medicine* 16, 9: 977–86.

Chapter 6

Researching the people's health

Dilemmas and opportunities for social scientists

Gareth Williams and Jennie Popay

INTRODUCTION

In the 1974 reorganization of the National Health Service (NHS), public health was killed off and replaced by community medicine (Jefferys 1986). Apparently, the problems of poverty and squalor, with which public health had wrestled (alongside others) since the nineteenth century, had been vanquished. All that was left, we were led to believe, was illness produced by the irresponsible acts of misinformed individuals. Cancer, heart disease, stroke, and bronchitis could be eliminated by the persistent application of educational messages directed at behavioural change. This new orthodoxy left little for community physicians to do other than advise 'the community', or individuals within the community, on good and bad 'lifestyles', and 'manage' health care. These principles – personal responsibility for health and the efficient management of health care – have solidified into the twin pillars upon which British health policy in the 1980s and 1990s has been based.

No sooner had community medicine been born, however, than the foundations of the new consensus which had produced it began to crack. A number of health problems emerged which clearly required more from public health than efficient management and health education. The dawning awareness of the distinct nature of health problems in the late twentieth century – notably the increasing prevalence of chronic illness – was paralleled by a recognition that these health problems were linked to a number of social and demographic factors. Amongst these are de-industrialization, insecurity of work and employment, the ageing population, the persistence of inequalities in living standards and health within affluent societies, and the consequences of environmental damage (Ashton and Seymour 1988). In response a new public health movement has developed, encompassing three important elements: first, a focus on the dangerousness of the physical and social environment; second, acknowledgement of the need to encourage the active participation of individuals and communities; and, third, recognition of the need to manufacture the collaboration of different sectors within society. These developments have been further encouraged by the World Health Organization's Health for All 2000 initiative (World Health Organization 1985). By the start of the 1990s the 'new public health' had become very much part of mainstream thinking (Acheson 1988; Porter and Porter 1990; Lancet 1991). Although the standard view of the new public health is that it is a radical response to the effects of social deregulation, it can also be seen as opening up spaces for new forms of surveillance and control by the State and its agents (Armstrong 1993)

Alongside the new public health movement and of immediate significance to it, a number of prominent political initiatives have been developed. In the last two years there have been White Papers on the hospital service and on community care (Department of Health 1989a, 1989b), the recommendations of which have now been enshrined in the NHS and Community Care Act 1991. Included within the provisions of this Act is the statutory requirement now placed upon district health authorities (DHAs) to assess the health needs of their resident populations – a process which must now explicitly include an enlarged perspective on researching the people's health (National Health Service Management Executive 1991). In addition, the government has also published a consultative document, followed by another White Paper, *The Health of the Nation* (Department of Health 1991a; Secretary of State for Health 1992) which, though conveniently failing to address the issue of class inequalities, has provided the opportunity for others to renew the debate about inequality and poverty (Smith and Egger 1993).

The new agenda that is being fashioned for public health has an important research component, and this contains space for social scientists of various hues. In trying to operate in this new space, however, they will face both opportunities and dilemmas. Social science could make a significant contribution to the understanding of the genesis and development of a whole range of health problems which are resistant to traditional epidemiological and public health methods. However, the dilemmas are several and perhaps familiar. Social scientists will have to resist the definition of their role coming from other actors in the arena – particularly, though not exclusively, medicine. They will have to think carefully about the extent and nature of their involvement in policy issues and their relationship to the values which different policies contain.

The dilemmas are brought sharply into focus in a recent document on assessing health needs from the National Health Service Management Executive (NHSME) DHA project. Here health needs are defined as the 'ability to benefit' from health care. The DHA project team takes a 'hybrid approach' to health needs assessment, proposing two strategies for the development of this approach: first, a methodology derived from 'a combined epidemiology and health economics standpoint', and, second, 'a pragmatic approach blurring the distinction between need and demand and between science and opinion, but which is available to help decision-making in the short term' (National Health Service Management Executive 1991: 3). In dichotomizing methodology in this way, the authors of this document reproduce the conventional distinction between the scientific and the non-scientific, between issues of objective need and clinical quality on the one hand, and matters of opinion or preference and non-clinical quality issues on the other.

In this paper we argue that the contribution of social science to health needs assessment and the wider agenda of public health research is fourfold. First, the alteration in the disease burden, and the growing importance of chronic illness and disablement, have revealed the limitations of classic epidemiology. The complex patterns of causes and consequences of chronic illness require that the 'methodology for the strict approach' to health-needs assessment consists of more than epidemiology and economics, and that the principal means of researching the people's health move beyond traditional epidemiology. Second, we argue that what the NHSME refers to as the blurred area between science and opinion is the *terra firma* of social science, particularly of sociology. Third, we contend that it will be necessary to apply the scientific requirements of research in this borderland if 'listening to local voices' and the 'corporate approach' to needs assessment are to be anything other than a genuflexion to the notion of participation and partnership. In the conclusion we suggest that, in addition to adding to knowledge, social science has an important role to play in facilitating the effective dissemination and use of the information it generates.

LIMITS TO EPIDEMIOLOGY

Epidemiology developed out of the confrontation of society with the major infectious diseases that followed the processes of industrialization and urbanization in the nineteenth century. There are many definitions of epidemiology. One of the more liberal tells us: 'Epidemiology is the branch of medical science that is concerned with studying the health of human communities' (Wood and Badley 1986: 59). This definition places the close relationship between epidemiology and community or public health firmly in the foreground. However, exclusion of things other than medical science from this definition, serves to expunge prematurely many activities which can contribute to understanding. The analytical and methodological problems raised by food-borne infections, environmental pollutants, HIV and AIDS, and many chronic and degenerative diseases, have highlighted the limits to traditional epidemiological models. These rest upon quasi-unifactorial models of aetiology and take ascertainment of cases of disease, rather than what happens after it, as their end-point (World Health Organization 1980).

These limitations have been most evident in relation to the epidemiology of chronic disease. In such a situation there may be no single, identifiable cause, the 'at risk' groups may be difficult to define and sample, the time-scale of symptom development is typically extended, the clinical outcome of the disease varies between individuals with the same disorder, and the outcome for the patient in terms of functional status can vary considerably even where the disease follows the same course. In short, there are three major problems posed for epidemiology by the preponderance of chronic disease: the problems of origin, prevalence and outcome.

Identifying the origins of disease

The problems posed for epidemiology in modelling the origins or causes of disease are perhaps seen most graphically in the case of coronary heart disease (CHD). Not only are the purported causes of CHD themselves multiple, posing complex questions about interactive effects at cellular, individual and social levels, but the relationship between these factors and the variables they are alleged to explain is highly uncertain. Studies of 'risk factors' for heart disease and heart attack, show that taken together these factors explain only small proportions of the variance (Marmot 1976). Moreover, not only is there debate over the nature and status of particular factors; there is disagreement over the explanatory frameworks within which the factors are defined (ibid. 1976). In these circumstances it is not easy either to confirm or to refute a particular theoretical proposition.

Epidemiology has difficulty in conceptualizing behavioural and social factors such as class, diet and stress, because they are not easily reducible to simple, unitary variables. If stress is equated with a simple life-event score, class with occupation, and diet with the type of fat used on bread, it is scarcely surprising that there is a large proportion of variance unexplained. Moreover, there is a sense in which epidemiologists, in their desire to be 'scientific' have felt uneasy about confronting directly such strongly evaluative problems as poverty and inequality.

Case ascertainment and prevalence

Ascertaining cases of disease and establishing prevalence are especially problematic in relation to HIV and AIDS and other conditions which are particularly common within population groups one way or another at the margins of society, and where identifying markers for 'at risk' status involve obtaining details of behaviour and lifestyle. In such situations the population or universe may be extremely variable, questions may be raised about the representativeness of those sampled, and response rates may be very low. In such contexts the need for a much broader definition of the appropriate disciplinary input to public health research becomes critical. Not only are traditional models of disease causation inadequate, as in CHD, but so also are traditional types of data and methods of data collection.

In the field of HIV and AIDS, for example, a great deal of thought has been given to the innovative use of qualitative methods of data collection, such as diaries, in-depth interviewing, and participant observation (McKeganey *et al.* 1990). These methods are part of the stock-in-trade of the social sciences. Issues to do with recall of information about personal behaviour, how to generate a sample, and how to ensure an adequate response rate from groups of people who have good reason to feel suspicious of official studies, raise major problems for traditional epidemiological studies of the health of population groups.

Understanding the consequences of disease

The third major problem for epidemiology is that it is dealing for the most part with diseases in which mortality is less important than morbidity, and in which incidence is relatively low and prevalence is relatively high. Heart disease, arthritis, stroke, bronchitis, asthma are conditions which, regardless of their capacity to cause death, are disabling.

The problem then becomes one of knowing what we should be establishing as prevalent. Clearly, for most purposes the issue is not about symptoms of disease, but rather the prevalence of the disabling consequences of the disease which may give rise to the need for different kinds of health and social care. Once disabling consequences become the focus, then any analysis confronts the fact that the severity of disability does not have a simple one-to-one relationship with the severity of the disease. Rather, it is the product of an interaction between the disease and a variety of psychological, social and economic factors.

The need to define disablement more systematically for both clinical and epidemiological purposes has been most rigorously argued by the WHO (World Health Organization 1980). Here impairment, disability and handicap were identified as representing different planes of experience which, taken together, constitute the 'consequences of disease'. The concept which relates most closely to the assessment of health needs is that of handicap. This represents the interaction between individuals and social circumstances. It is defined as 'a disadvantage for a given individual, resulting from an impairment or disability, that limits or prevents the fulfilment of a role that is normal (depending on age, sex, and social and cultural factors) for that individual' (WHO 1980: 29).

The concept of handicap relates to the experiences of chronically ill people in their daily lives, and, by definition, it requires us to move beyond biomedical parameters to encompass social and cultural factors. From the point of view of the assessment of health needs, an epidemiology of chronic disease must include some assessment of the impact of disease on the quality of everyday life. The development of measures to take account of this have long been of concern in clinical and rehabilitation medicine, and are increasingly being discussed within mainstream health services research (Bowling 1993)

The difficulty in identifying meaningful risk factors for CHD, the elusiveness of the populations studied for HIV transmission, and the difficulties of conceptualizing and measuring disablement point to the critical role the social sciences have to play within the development of a science adequate to the new agenda for researching the people's health. The kinds of methodological problems that we have discussed in outline here show how vital it is to apply the 'sociological imagination' to health needs assessment in particular and to public health research in general.

What all this leads us to believe is that the methodology for health needs assessment must depart from rigid adherence to classic models of epidemiology and health economics. Many public health problems, because of the social and behavioural factors which influence their origins and their effects, require much more flexible definitions of research, science and data.

RESEARCH IN THE BORDERLANDS BETWEEN SCIENCE AND OPINION

In recent years there has been growing interest in improving the communications between lay people and professionals in situations where a health problem is ill-defined. The corporate approach to health needs assessment put forward by the NHSME clearly wishes to extend this so as to bring together a whole range of different interests (lay, medical, local authority, voluntary sector) in dealing with the assessment of complex health and health care problems.

Such research inhabits the borderlands between science and opinion, and it is here that we would locate the second major niche for social science. Through an examination of the response to an environmental health hazard – the Camelford incident – we want to develop three points. First, we argue that research into lay perspectives on health needs and public health issues in general is more problematic than the NHSME appears to realize when it refers to this as the 'pragmatic' approach to needs assessment. Second, we argue that simply because research in these borderlands does not fit the methodology of the strict approach to needs assessment described by the NHSME, this does not release us from the obligation to study these issues rigorously in a 'scientific' manner. Third, we suggest that social science has an important contribution to make to this endeavour.

Local voices in the Lowermoor water incident

On 6 July 1988, a lorry-driver accidentally tipped twenty tonnes of aluminium sulphate solution into the water tank supplying the Lowermoor waterworks, which serves the residents of Camelford and the surrounding area in north Cornwall. This episode has been the subject of two reports from an expert committee, the Lowermoor Incident Health Advisory Group, chaired by Dame Barbara Clayton, a well-respected chemical pathologist (Cornwall and Isles of Scilly Health Authority 1989; Department of Health 1991b). In addition to Barbara Clayton, the group consisted of a neurochemical pathologist, the chief scientist of the Water Research Centre, and a professor of epidemiology.

Nobody now disputes the immediate effects, which, according to the Clayton Report, included: 'nausea, vomiting, diarrhoea, headaches, fatigue, itching skin, rashes, sore eyes, and mouth ulcers'. The Report goes on to register that some people felt 'generally unwell' while others complained of 'aches and pains'. The Report notes the difficulty in assessing the reliability and significance of such reports, and points out that consultation patterns with local general practitioners did not show any increase in the month following the incident.

The Clayton Committee also received information from the Camelford Scientific Advisory Panel (CSAP), a local voluntary group set up to monitor the matter. The CSAP produced its own questionnaire, which was completed by 432 people between mid-July and mid-August. The most commonly reported complaints were similar to those which the official group had identified in its independent investigations. The Clayton Committee noted, however, that detailed analysis of the CSAP information was not appropriate because of the unrepresentative, self-selected nature of the sample. Nonetheless, they judged that 'many of the early symptoms reported to CSAP and at our meeting in Camelford can be attributed to the incident' (Cornwall and Isles of Scilly Health Authority 1989: 3).

The disagreement between the Clayton Report and local residents stemmed from the facts about the 'delayed or persistent effects' of the incident. The Report notes that the health authority has compiled a register of people complaining about symptoms occurring or persisting long after the incident. At the time the report was written in July 1989 there were 280 people on the register.

In its examination the official group studied the concentration of a variety of contaminants in relation to European Community standards. For lead, zinc, copper and sulphate, they concluded that the amounts likely to have been absorbed, even on a worst-case assumption, would have no long-lasting effects on the health of the population. In relation to aluminium, the major pollutant, and in view of the complaints of memory loss and the recent attention given to the possibility of a link between aluminium and Alzheimer's disease, the report presents its summary of evidence regarding the dietary sources, metabolism and toxicology of aluminium. However, they still concluded that any ill-health caused by the aluminium was temporary.

Although they claimed to refute the linkage of the contamination and long-term health effects, they clearly felt obliged to offer some explanation and concluded: 'In our view it is not possible to attribute the very real current health complaints to the toxic effects of the incident, except inasmuch as they are the consequence of the sustained anxiety naturally felt by many people' (ibid.: 14); anxiety which they saw as being fuelled by irresponsible reporting in the media.

The response to the Clayton Report

The press and other media have played a major role in publicizing the Camelford incident and in discussing points of view which are opposed to the conclusions and recommendations of the Clayton Committee. People continue to complain of symptoms of malaise, and in particular problems with memory and other aspects of cognitive functioning. In view of the continuing commotion, a special conference was convened by the Cornwall and Isles of Scilly Health Authority in February 1990 (Cornwall and Isles of Scilly Health Authority 1990). Three papers presented at the conference fuelled the debate: a clinical biochemist found high concentrations of aluminium in blood samples one year after the incident; a neuropsychologist reported evidence 'consistent with the effects of minor brain injury'; and a clinical psychologist discovered significant memory defects. The fact that the conference report did not get published until the findings were leaked to the press, almost six months after the conference met, led some people to feel that something was being hidden.

Throughout the period since July 1988 to now, organized opposition to the official view has been articulated by local people in the Lowermoor Support Group and the CSAP. The latter, according to one report, is 'an *ad hoc* group of people living in the area who have academic or campaigning skills. It includes Liz Sigmund, a veteran of the campaign against chemical weapons, Dr Newman (a local GP who has himself experienced problems with memory), and Doug Cross, an environmental consultant' (Kennedy 1990: 4).

The Department of Health reacted to the accusations by local residents and the media which had given them a platform. The Junior Health Minister, Stephen Dorrell, reacted first in a letter to the *Guardian*, where he criticized the newspaper for:

> Grossly misrepresent(ing) the properly cautious conclusions of the (Clayton) report, based as it was on a detailed and thorough assessment of the scientific data available. No more and no less would be expected from a group of truly independent and distinguished scientists, who are acknowledged experts in the relevant fields.
>
> (Dorrell 1990)

Then, in a parliamentary reply, the critics of the Report resident in Camelford were characterized as: 'malicious people, down there stirring things up, and worrying people for their own short-term gains' (Phillips 1990: 19). The decision that the Clayton Committee was to be reconvened, with the same membership, to consider the matter again, was greeted with dismay by local residents and their supporters. Liz Sigmund of the CSAP was quoted in the newspapers as saying: 'One whitewash will be followed by another, unless they are all prepared to admit they were wrong, which seems highly unlikely' (Brown 1990: 3).

From the point of view of these remarks, such anxieties seem to have been well founded. The second Clayton Report (Department of Health 1991b) broadly reiterated its conclusions that there was no evidence that the ailments local people had attributed to the accident were caused by toxic water. The chief medical officer insisted that Clayton and her colleagues 'have again carried out a difficult task with sensitivity and integrity' (Calman 1991).

SOCIAL SCIENCE AND THE HEALTH OF COMMUNITIES

The incident at Camelford, and the context in which it took place, illustrate two points relevant to the agenda for public health and health needs assessment research. First, and contrary to the NHSME's separation of a strict methodology from something more opinionated, the pursuit of knowledge is never completely divorced from interests (Habermas 1978). The ability to claim, against the claims of others, that one's knowledge is valid is a very powerful claim. However, in relation to real causes of public ill-health, the status of the evidence available makes it extremely difficult to apply the 'methodology for the strict approach'.

Second, the incident is a good example of the way in which real-life public health issues exist in a murky borderland between science and opinion. The corporate approach to the assessment of health needs will bring together people with different opinions and different world-views. As the Camelford example illustrates, however, the problem is one of mediating not just between lay and professional people, but also between different kinds of professionals, and between a variety of media and political interests. There is no easy way of resolving the conflicts that will inevitably surface, but social science can provide a framework for working with such conflict productively. This framework, however, does not involve 'unscientific' activity that can be done without attention to theory, method and the broader context of political and economic interests.

Social scientists have long worked with the understanding that the knowledge they produce is value-laden, and have long since ceased to see their work in terms of opposition between science and opinion, between rationality and irrationality, passion and logic, and commitment and detachment. Social scientists recognize that in studying the 'life-world' of individuals or the 'culture' of social agencies, a variety of rationalities and alternative discourses will be revealed. Within each of these, the actors involved will be operating with different criteria not only of validity, but of legitimacy and authenticity (Habermas 1984). This means that conflicts over definition are an intrinsic part of the business of a corporate approach to public health issues. In short, social science is ideally placed, both because of the heterogeneity of its theoretical perspectives and by virtue of its pluralistic approach to methods, to make a contribution to researching these issues and informing decision-making in relation to them.

A MULTITUDE OF VOICES REQUIRES A PLURALITY OF PERSPECTIVES

Social science has a variety of different methodological tools available to research the borderlands between science and opinion: participant observation, intensive interviewing, ethnography and case study. Such methods are often regarded as 'unreliable' when compared with traditional epidemiological methods because of their unstructured and relatively uncontrolled nature. However, their 'unreliability' relative to the 'gold standard' of the randomized controlled trial is hardly a limitation – and indeed may be seen as a strength – when the object is an investigation in a 'naturally-occurring' situation (Pope and Mays 1993). Moreover, in circumstances where the definition of the problems is potentially contested and where the population to be sampled is uncertain, these 'unreliable' methods are precisely those required to make sense of the situation. In addition – and in view of the expressed desire in the new public health and health needs assessment to encourage community and lay participation and to seek partnerships between different sectors – these methods actually encourage participation and tap the respondents' own points of view.

The data derived through these methods cannot, of course, be judged according to the same criteria as those applied to an epidemiological survey. But this does not mean that they are, *ipso facto*, unreliable or invalid; it means that they have to be appraised and evaluated in terms of different criteria. The kinds of generalization that one can make from a case study are inevitably different from those that one can make from a sample survey, but they are no less powerful (Mitchell 1983). The kinds of problem faced by public health research in general and health needs assessment in particular require flexibility and imagination in the use of methods. This does not mean reducing science to 'chatting to the locals', or indeed to 'the experts'. It means that discovering and interpreting alternative perspectives require a different kind of science. It is the dawning realization of this in some settings that has led people to bring a variety of sociological techniques and approaches into what is referred to as 'Rapid Appraisal' (see Chapter 4).

The social sciences are also equipped to enter this borderland because of the nature of the theoretical perspectives and concepts they are accustomed to using. Debate over the meaning and empirical application of concepts like power, community, interest, conflict, cooperation, profession, rationality, and so on, are part of the stock-in-trade of sociologists. While theoretical discussion of such concepts may be viewed by some as a form of navel-gazing, such conceptual understanding is indispensable to the public health research agenda. This is particularly so at a time when the traditional patterns of authority and deference between patients and doctors, between accountants and scientists and between managers and consultants are breaking down (Gabe *et al.* 1994).

For those who remain unconvinced, and would like to remain safe within the shell of normal science, it is perhaps necessary to emphasize that what we have written is less a bid for a piece of future action and more a reference to where we already are. The debate over the new public health, and the concern to define the best approach to health needs assessment, are just one example of the way in which relations between lay people, different occupational groups, civil society, and the State are changing. The community-health movement, the toxic-waste movement, and other manifestations of public participation, point to a growing dissatisfaction both with the elitism of expert knowledge and with exclusion from effective democratic activity (Williams and Popay 1994).

Corporate discussions about health needs assessment and other public health issues involve ethical and political challenges to those who make the environment 'unhealthy' and those who, in the past, have decided health care priorities. But they also carry with them an epistemological challenge to epidemiologists and other experts in public and environmental health, including managers. If health needs assessment and the NHSME's 'pragmatic approach' are to be more than a genuflexion to community concerns and intersectoral collaboration, effective methods for listening to the multitude of voices must be developed, and ways of creating a genuine synthesis of different interests and perspectives need to be set up.

Epidemiology cannot resolve the public health problems of everyday life by retiring into the epistemology of medicine. There is much talk nowadays about 'rapid epidemiological appraisal' and even 'rapid ethnographic appraisal'. Such work must involve a commitment to grasping the varying perspectives of all interested parties, and to confronting the issues of who controls both the findings of epidemiological research, and its conceptualization. To do this means facing up to disputes not just over the facts of a particular issue, but also over the criteria for what is to count as a fact; disagreement over understandings of cause and effect; and conflict based upon the different interests. The question is how to collect reliable information on different perspectives, and to examine the competing claims they make. Sociology is ideally placed to play a role in relation to these dilemmas.

CONCLUSIONS

We have pointed to some of the opportunities and dilemmas we believe presently face social science in relation to the new research agenda for public health and health needs assessment. Taking as our starting-point the most recent and much-discussed NHSME document on assessing health needs, we identified major areas of opportunity within both the NHSME's narrowly drawn 'strict approach' and the borderlands between science and opinion described as the 'corporate approach'. Any attempt by social scientists to make a case for their involvement in these areas can only be enhanced by the new thirst for information evident amongst health authorities. The renewed emphasis within the NHS in general, and public health in particular, on participation and partnership also holds out the prospect of exciting collaborative work which will serve to enlarge our understanding.

However, in seizing these opportunities, social scientists also have to face up to a number of difficult dilemmas. Some of these are long-standing. There is the problematic status of social science as a science, and the debate over the validity and reliability of social science data. These issues will not be finally resolved in this arena (if indeed they are resolved anywhere), but the involvement of social science in public health research and health needs assessment and the wider recognition of the value of this contribution, will serve to challenge the critics. The essentially political nature of many of the issues on the research agenda also presents dilemmas for those social scientists who venture into this terrain. What is important is that social scientists do not allow their work to be defined as inherently more political than the apparently value-free science of the 'strict approach'.

Finally, the sociological imagination has to operate with awareness of the role of structures in society, and this includes an understanding of the way in which they work in relation to the research it produces and the extent to which it succeeds in facilitating change in social organizations. Knowledge does not exist in a social and political void. One of the slightly naive assumptions about health care and health services is that change and improvement will follow from knowledge. This often leads to a failure to recognize that knowledge is also something that is constrained and produced by social structures. Such processes will have important implications for the fate of the veritable avalanche of information on health needs that is descending on to NHS purchasers and providers at the present time. If such information is to be used effectively to facilitate change, then the way it is collected must be linked to its possible uses, and the way in which it is used within the NHS must also be the subject of sustained study. Sociological understanding of power, conflict, discourse and interests can point to the complexities inherent in the process of change and help to identify the barriers. This is clearly of crucial importance if health services are really going to be driven by the knowledge derived from the assessment of health needs.

ACKNOWLEDGEMENTS

We are grateful to Rob Flynn, Neil McKeganey and Joel Richman for their helpful comments on earlier drafts.

REFERENCES

Acheson, D. (1988) *Public Health in England: The Report of the Committee of Inquiry into the Future of the Public Health Function*, Cm 289, London: HMSO.

Armstrong, D. (1993) 'Public health spaces and the fabrication of identity', *Sociology* 27: 393–410.

Ashton, J., and Seymour, H. (1988) *The New Public Health*, Milton Keynes: Open University Press.

Bowling, A. (1993) *Measuring Health: A Review of Quality of Life Measurement Scales*, Buckingham: Open University Press.

Brown, P. (1990) 'Water poisoning inquiry reopens at Camelford', *The Guardian*, 16 October.

Calman, K. (1991) 'Camelford report's clear lines of inquiry' (letter) *The Guardian*, 12 November.

Cornwall and Isles of Scilly Health Authority (1989) *Water Pollution at Lowermoor, North Cornwall: Report of the Lowermoor Incident Health Advisory Group*, Truro: Cornwall and Isles of Scilly District Health Authority.

—— (1990) *Lowermoor Water Incident*, Proceedings of the conference held on 3 February 1990 at the postgraduate centre, Royal Cornwall Hospital, Treliske, Truro, Truro: Cornwall and Isles of Scilly Health Authority.

Department of Health (1989a) *Working for Patients*, London: HMSO.

—— (1989b) *Caring for People: Community Care in the Next Decade and Beyond*, London: HMSO.

—— (1991a) *The Health of the Nation*, London: HMSO.

—— (1991b) *Water Pollution at Lowermoor, North Cornwall: Second Report of the Lowermoor Incident Health Advisory Group*, London: HMSO.

Dorrell, S. (1990) 'Government concern over the suffering in Camelford' (letter), *The Guardian*, 27 July.

Gabe, J., Kelleher, D., and Williams, G., eds (1994) *Challenging Medicine*, London: Routledge.

Habermas, J. (1978) *Knowledge and Human Interests*, London: Heinemann.

—— (1984) *The Theory of Communicative Action*, Volume 1: *Reason and the Rationalization of Society*, trans. Thomas McCarthy, Boston, Mass.: Beacon Press.

Jefferys, M. (1986) 'The transition from public health to community medicine; the evolution and execution of a policy for occupational transformation', *Bulletin for the Social History of Medicine* 39: 47–63.

Kennedy, M. (1990) 'Water blunder turned the good life sour', *The Guardian*, 11 June.

Lancet (1991) 'What's new in public health' (editorial), *The Lancet* 337: 1381–2.

McKeganey, N., Barnard, M., and Bloor, M. (1990) 'A comparison of HIV-related risk behaviour and risk reduction between female street-working prostitutes and male rent boys in Glasgow', *Sociology of Health and Illness* 12: 274–92.

Marmot, M. (1976) 'Facts, opinions, and *affaires du coeur*', *American Journal of Epidemiology* 103: 519–26.

Mitchell, J.C. (1983) Case and situation analysis', *Sociological Review* 31: 187–211.

National Health Service Management Executive (1991) *Assessing Health Care Needs: a NHS Project Discussion Paper*, London: National Health Service Management Executive.

Phillips, M. (1990) 'The seeping sickness of Camelford', *The Guardian*, 26 October.

Pope, C., and Mays, N. (1993) 'Opening the black box: an encounter in the corridors of health services research', *British Medical Journal* 306: 315–18.

Porter, D. and Porter, R. (1990) 'The ghost of Edwin Chadwick', *British Medical Journal* 301: 252.

Secretary of State for Health (1992) *The Health of the Nation: A Strategy for Health in England*, Cm 1986, London: HMSO.

Smith, G. Davey, and Egger, M. (1993) 'Socio-economic differentials in wealth and health', *British Medical Journal* 307: 1085–6.

Williams, G., and Popay, J. (1994) 'Lay knowledge and the privilege of experience', in Gabe, J., Kelleher, D., and Williams, G., eds, *Challenging Medicine*, London: Routledge.

Wood, P.H.N., and Badley, E.M. (1986) 'Epidemiology of individual rheumatic disorders', in Scott, J.T., ed., *Copeman's Textbook of the Rheumatic Diseases*, 6th edn, London: Churchill Livingstone.

World Health Organization (1980) *International Classification of Impairments, Disabilities, and Handicaps: A Manual Relating to the Consequences of Disease*, Geneva: World Health Organization.

—— (1985) *Targets for Health for All*, Copenhagen: World Health Organization.

Chapter 7

'It's like teaching your child to swim in a pool full of alligators'

Lay voices and professional research on child accidents

Cathie Rice, Helen Roberts, Susan J. Smith and Carol Bryce

INTRODUCTION

Much of the policy debate on risk management relies on the formula that the 'experts' will tell you what the real dangers are and how to reduce them. Frequently, the experts' messages give reassurance that anxieties are ill-founded. Practical advice on risk reduction tends to require changes in the behaviour of potential victims, rather than in those who produce the risk. Nowhere is this more the case than in the field of child safety. Children must be taught to shout 'No' and run from danger; they must be taught never to cross a road if a car is coming and never to cross between parked cars; they must be taught of stranger danger, and danger in the home.

According to this perspective, not only are children inclined to take risks which endanger their own health, but mothers are depicted as presenting a danger to their children, an observation which has been made in other contexts (Graham 1982). Safety is one of the many areas of child health where mothers are given little credit when things go right but are inclined to be blamed when they go wrong. As a poster (now, happily, withdrawn) from a leading safety organization, intended to encourage parents to pick up their children from school helpfully put it, 'Some parents just don't care.'

This chapter describes some of the background issues, social context and social relationships embedded in a study of child accidents and the maintenance of safety which ran alongside a parents' action group on child safety in Corkerhill, a housing estate in Glasgow. The study explored safety as a social value.

CORKERHILL: THE SETTING AND THE CONTEXT

Corkerhill is a housing scheme in the south of Glasgow. Its boundaries are a busy main road, a railway with an unattended station, a river and an area of parkland. It has around 580 dwellings, a predominantly social class IV/V population, and high unemployment. There is low access to personal transport, low home-ownership, and over one-third of households with children are headed by a lone parent.

To describe Corkerhill in terms of socio-economic indicators is misleading; the people who live there are not merely 'objects' of professional concern. Within the relatively narrow parameters open to them, repeated attempts are made by residents to shape and improve their lives and those of their children, and to widen the arena within which they can move and operate. They have been involved in a number of public health issues and met with some considerable success.

We were not working in Corkerhill because of its 'accidentogenic' properties. We were working there because we were invited in, and because the community had an agenda which coincided, to a certain extent, with ours. As it turned out, the accident admission rates for Corkerhill are rather higher than those for similar neighbourhood types in Glasgow, and over twice as high as those for the city as a whole.

A large number of local people were involved in this work, some directly, others indirectly. At times, a substantial minority of the community would be packed into the cramped quarters of the local community 'shop' – a meeting-room – to discuss issues arising from the study or the associated campaign. Inevitably, there was a small core group of people with whom we worked closely. These were Cathie Rice, Betty Campbell and Walter Morrison. At the time, Cathie Rice was chair of Corkerhill Community Council (a non-political tier of local government in Scotland whose role is to identify the needs of their community and to make these views known to the local and public authorities). She is the mother of three children, the youngest born at the time the study was being planned. Betty Campbell, who has now taken on the chair of the community council, is a mother of adult children and a grandmother. Her husband was murdered in an unprovoked attack in the locality not long before this work started. Walter Morrison is a father of adult children, and has for many years been the secretary of the Corkerhill community council. He has fought hard for his community in dozens of battles. The title of this chapter is a phrase of his. None of the people described here is active in party politics. The local community, their needs, their families, their neighbours and their children are the driving force behind their activity.

The community council has been concerned with a variety of safety issues over many years. Our research coincided with a period of renewed vigour in their work on child-safety issues at the local level. The research therefore ran alongside, informed and was informed by a parents' action campaign around accident reduction and child safety.

No doubt there is more than one community story of our research. The one which follows was written by Cathie Rice. A housewife and mother, and chair of the community council at the time the work described here was carried out, she has since been employed on a safety project in a community close to Corkerhill.

THE CORKERHILL STUDY: A COMMUNITY VIEW

When communities find themselves labelled 'areas of deprivation, social class IV/V', and so on, it might seem normal to expect that any proposed research into 'what ails us' would be welcomed. The reality is somewhat different. In common with community organizations elsewhere, we in Corkerhill do of course recognize that the professional research body may be able to take information through doors which the community cannot open, but we have learned to be cautious, if not downright suspicious, of those who would 'assist' us in this way.

Too often we have been subjected to the 'goldfish bowl' approach to research. We have been researched upon. The researcher selects the topic, studies his subject and returns to the lofty towers of academia leaving a bemused community who very soon realize that they have gained nothing from the experience. Despite this apparent cynicism, not only do we recognize the need for good research and the powerful potential it has, but we are confident enough to believe that we have a contribution to make to it.

Community approach

Most community groups believe that the only positive approach to local issues is from the bottom up. This is not simply because we see ourselves as squarely at the bottom of the social scale but because living daily with the problems of poverty, poor housing, unemployment and raising children in what can only be described as a hostile environment, we have our own 'expertise'.

If community research is to be meaningful it must be carried out with the full cooperation of the community in partnership with the academics. It must also address issues which are identified as priorities by local people. Our experience has been that the most successful campaigns have been those initiated by tenants themselves. In recent years we have successfully campaigned against the use of chemicals in the treatment of dampness in our houses and the treatment of children who have sustained needlestick injury. These issues were brought to our attention by local residents, and consequently they themselves were willing to support our efforts to bring about change.

Corkerhill and public health research

Around the time of these local campaigns we made contact with Helen Roberts who was then at Glasgow University. We wanted to ask if she and her colleagues would help us with some work on the connection between our children's asthma, damp housing and the chemicals used to treat the mould in our houses. She was not able to help us with this herself, but put us in touch with Sonja Hunt, who with her colleagues Claudia Martin and Steve Platt, had worked on damp housing (Martin *et al.* 1987). As part of another project, some local mothers took part in a video compiled by her colleague David Stone. This was aimed at doctors and health visitors and it was hoped it would help them understand not only the easily identifiable effects of poverty and bad housing on the health of their patients, but perhaps the less readily accepted effects of stress on these women too (Stone with Roberts 1992).

Helen visited Corkerhill on many occasions over a fairly long period of time and was often present during our lengthy discussions about issues of importance to the community. Thus a level of communication and trust was built. It was clear that Helen and her colleagues Carol Bryce and Susan Smith believed in a collaborative approach to working with local people. In this sense, the normal way of going about things was reversed. We involved Helen Roberts and Susan Smith in work that was relevant to our community, rather than them coming to us with a bright idea.

The issue of child safety was raised by local parents and was a natural progression from work which had been undertaken by the community council's members. We had already done work related to safety, although we probably wouldn't have called it 'work'. It *was* hard work, but it is the kind of daily struggle which we and people in communities like ours expect to engage in on a daily basis. We had campaigned, for instance, for a better play area. We had strongly opposed a new road planned to cross the back of our community, cutting us off from our one local amenity, an area of beautiful woodland and countryside containing the world-famous Burrell art collection. The choice had been: did the nearby golf club get cut off by the road, or did we? We did, but as some consolation for daily attendance at the public inquiry over six weeks, we were offered a new play park. We had campaigned, with some success, against the use of chemicals to treat mould in our houses, and had carried out a survey ourselves to look at what people believe to be the health effects on themselves, their children and their household pets of these chemicals. This resulted in a 'Damphouse Inquiry' which we held in the community shop, chaired by a local Justice of the Peace (JP) and with attendance invited (and in some cases, taken up) by relevant local authority departments.

After a number of needlestick injuries to children in the neighbourhood as a result of needles left around by drug users, we realized that our local accident and emergency department did not have ready supplies of immunoglobin. It had to be obtained on a named-patient basis from the regional blood transfusion service. Most of us in Corkerhill do not have access to a private car, so this involved not only the anxiety of a day's wait for treatment, but the cost in time and money of a second bus or taxi ride to the hospital after the initial visit. We raised our concerns with the local health promotion department with little success. They were friendly, but felt that their role was to 'reassure' us that the dangers from needlestick injuries were exaggerated (and, by the by, we would be better off giving up smoking to protect our children). Our next port of call was the district council's management committee, which served the south-west area in Glasgow. From there we were directed to the sub-committee on drug misuse. A letter from the Director of Public Health followed this meeting. He assured us he would deal with it. Getting things done, and being heard, as we were by the Director of Public Health, is important. Having some successes is vital in maintaining the momentum to continue to struggle for a healthier, safer environment for our children and ourselves. This kind of constructive response to an issue highlighted by the community is very welcome, if unusual.

When community groups from similar types of area, be they in Glasgow, Manchester, Liverpool or elsewhere, have met there has been instant recognition of problems, and the types of responses given by professionals to those problems. Dampness could provoke responses such as 'These people make their homes damp so they can get a house near their mum', 'It's not dampness pet – it's condensation. Burn all your fires, keep all of your windows open during the day, don't wash clothes, make soup, or boil too many kettles. Oh, and try not to breathe too hard in the bedroom.' Almost funny if you don't consider childhood asthma, ruined clothes, furniture and lives. Then there is the response of those who would like to be 'pals'. They would speak a little more loudly, more slowly, with a few slang words here or there. Or the paternalistic response such as the one we had from the roads department offering to educate us. After a spate of accidents to children, we had written to them with some constructive suggestions about making local roads safer. The response was: "I do not see much scope for removing the inherent danger of parked vehicles since these most probably belong to residents. Barrier rails would not be practical since drivers require access to the footway . . . . I feel therefore, that the best means of addressing the situation is to increase parental awareness of the need to supervise young children and to teach them about the dangers of playing near traffic. To that end, Road Safety staff will be contacting you . . . . Thank you for your interest and concern for road safety . . .'

As community representatives, we have expressed in many forums the view that communities have their own expertise to offer and that, important though education is, it cannot counter the effects of poverty and a dangerous environment. The research would ask the community to prove this expertise.

I speak only for myself when I confess to a few moments' trepidation. What if no one took part? What if we were wrong and the educationalists had it right all along?

The research process

For the project to be a success, we needed the cooperation of all the residents in the area, especially the parents. During the initial round of group interviews we not only found to our relief that parents were happy to take part in the process, but during the course of the discussions it emerged that there were common beliefs in our own coping abilities, and about the effects of living in an unhealthy environment. There was also a hope (perhaps an over-optimistic one) that by taking part in this exercise we could change some of the opinions held by many so-called experts, particularly those who seem to believe that education is all that is needed to ensure the well-being of our children. 'Because I do not have safety equipment for my child does not mean that I need to be educated in the fact that such equipment exists – I simply do not have the money to purchase it.'

These group sessions did much to confirm our belief that the risk of accidents to our children is greatly increased by the fact that we live in an environment which is at best not child-friendly – *not* because we as parents are somehow more remiss than our more affluent contemporaries in the up-market areas of Glasgow. The meetings were also in their way social events. Glaswegians will always welcome a visitor with a cup of tea and a chat, and humour was never far away. They showed too that rather than mourn community spirit, there is much to gain from providing opportunities to rekindle it.

The outcome

Although local residents did not act as interviewers themselves, they played an important role in helping to devise the survey. They also helped to arrange interviews and generally became the linchpin between the researchers and the community. The results of this work have served to give a stronger voice to this community, because we can support our claims with statistical evidence for which we are grateful to Helen, Susan and Carol, and their colleagues.

Perhaps it was testament to this community's desire to work for change that so much detailed information was given. Any parent will speak freely about the dangers of the environment, traffic routes and so on. 'Home' creates images of safety, warmth and care. Housing in Corkerhill, with its open verandas, live sockets, easily opened windows, and fungi on walls, denies our children a safe place to live. Unemployment and poverty prevent parents from making changes. It would seem that priorities within Corkerhill have come full circle, with housing firmly as the priority.

During the course of the work, Helen Roberts introduced us to Professor Leif Svanström from the Karolinska Institute at the University of Stockholm, whose department has a strong interest in community safety and is a World Health Organization (WHO) collaborating centre on Safe Communities. He visited us, and encouraged us to apply for Safe Community status. With some reservations, we did so (Morrison *et al.* 1992). Would this just be a certificate on the wall? Would it do anything to make the community safer? We were given Safe Community status, and have had many visitors from all over the world, ranging from police officers and public health physicians to road engineers and paediatricians. They do not come to admire all the changes that have been made in the community – there have been some, but few. They come because they have heard that we have a vision of what a safe community could be like, and what we need to do to achieve that. We are frequently asked to talk about our work in Scotland, other parts of the UK, and further afield.

It would be relatively easy to measure physical change within a community. Sadly the roofs are still flat, the play area is still woefully inadequate and most of the other hazards are still there. But change is not measured only in these terms. This piece of work helped to increase the self-esteem of people within the community – it gave a voice to those who are often silent. It was a valued learning experience, which we would not have missed and for which we are grateful. We enjoyed it too. I found a distant relative and it helped me to get a job.

It is perhaps too soon to tell how significant this work will be in effecting change not only for this community but for similar areas throughout the country . . . . *will anyone listen*?

THE CORKERHILL STUDY: A RESEARCHER'S STORY

While charity advertisements might lead one to suppose that the greatest threat to a child's health is cancer or leukaemia, child accidents are the main cause of child death in the United Kingdom after the age of 1 and a considerable cause of morbidity in children and anxiety in their parents. Despite the fact that child death and injury from accidents are a major public health problem, there has until recently been remarkably little scientific research evaluating the relationship of safety education to child accidents and injuries (Towner *et al.* 1993). There is hardly any information on what safety measures people take, or what safety behaviours parents routinely practice (Worfwel and de Geus 1993). This neglect is especially alarming in the light of concerns about health inequalities, since not only are accidents a major problem, but they are a problem which disproportionately affects people living in poverty (Avery *et al.* 1990).

In spite of this lack of scientific endeavour, there can be little doubt that if there were not a very well-developed set of maternal (or parental) competencies in preventing child accidents, no child would make it to adulthood even if brought up under relatively safe and affluent conditions. In starting the research, the puzzle for us was not 'Why do child accidents happen?' but, rather, given the demonstrable risks built into Corkerhill's environment, how is it that most parents manage to keep their children safe most of the time?

While it has long been recognized by those working on occupational health and safety that many safety lessons must be learned from those who work in unsafe environments, and on the basis as much of the accidents which do not happen as of those that do, work on children and home accidents has much more frequently been based on a deficit model of educating individual children or individual parents (usually mothers) within individual families. In setting up our research, by contrast, we wanted to approach the problem in a way that would enable us to learn from what parents already know about keeping their children safe. Individual parents, knowing the dangers, can only respond by avoidance or protection. But their knowledge, when it informs policy, could be used to reduce external perils. It is not unusual in aviation and anaesthetics for safety practices to be based on averted accidents as well as on the accidents that happen. Could this kind of knowledge also be tapped in relation to child accidents?

People who live in a particular community, we hypothesized, are well placed to recognize dangers specific to that community and their own dwellings, and to advise on the reduction of these dangers. This is, ironically, especially true where risks are high and hazards are an everyday affair. The answers to a number of questions around child safety were, we felt, there to be uncovered, rather than 'discovered'. The local voices and the lay knowledge held the key, as they have to many health problems in the past, including in particular industrially related illnesses. The story of those working with (or widowed by) asbestos, who were convinced of the work link at an early stage, came well in advance of scientific work on mesothelioma. In the early 1950s, there was a pit disaster at Easington colliery in County Durham. Two rescue workers and eighty-one miners died. The men had suspected there was something wrong with the colliery months before. 'What's she like?' they would ask each other at shift change. 'As full of gas as a bottle of pop' was a reply (Oxford 1993: 5).

It is not surprising that people become aware of the risks and dangers around them. It would be strange if they did not. We believe that those living with the risks and dangers of a local community are likely to have much the kind of untapped knowledge that would help us better understand the studies of risk factors linking, for instance, accidents with lone parenthood, unemployment, low maternal age and overcrowding which have been frequently described but remain poorly explained (Wadsworth *et al.* 1983; Pless *et al.* 1989).

The project

The aims of the project were:

- to identify factors predisposing children to be at risk of, and protected from, accidents in the home and the wider environment;
- to investigate the strategies which families adopt to maintain safety,

and look at the ways in which safety-keeping is incorporated into routine family behaviour.

Our aim below is to write about the context and process of the research rather than the findings, which are described in detail elsewhere (Roberts *et al.* 1993, 1995; Bryce *et al.* 1993).

Research design

Our research design aimed to build on issues 'known' to the community. There were three parts to the study:

1. a series of group interviews designed to explore the salience of various issues around child safety to people in the community and to a group of professionals with responsibility for safety in the community
2. a household survey of all families in Corkerhill with a child aged 14 or under, and, in order to identify these families, a shorter screening survey of all households
3. case studies of successful and unsuccessful accident-prevention strategies, based on accidents and near misses identified during the survey.

In what ways were the lay voices heard?

Starting the research

Local people were involved in this research at its inception. Research agendas do not drop from the sky, and are frequently constrained by funding, political, policy and other considerations. At the time the work was set up, child accident research did not have the priority which subsequently resulted from the publication of *The Nation's Health* (Department of Health 1992). The research derived from anxieties parents felt about the safety of their children in Corkerhill, which went well beyond whether they would be run over by a car. As Cathie Rice has noted, the cold, damp housing had long been identified as a health hazard as well as a social disaster. The purchase and sale of drugs had resulted in needles being found in a number of closes (the common entrance halls to blocks of flats or tenements). A new road was about to be built cutting Corkerhill off from its one social amenity and along which a traffic flow of 40,000 vehicles a day would pass within twenty-five yards of the community's run-down children's playground.

As the community educated the researchers into the wide meanings which can be attached to child safety by those living in unsafe environments, the researchers were able to bring to the community understandings about the role of social epidemiology in describing and understanding patterns of accidents, and the ways in which these can be used. Links were forged with other institutions, people and countries, and the research became a way of validating locally much of what local people already 'knew' to be the case.

The first stage: the group interviews

We began with some work which involved group interviews with people living in different types of housing in Corkerhill, with a group of teenagers, and with a group of health professionals. The intention was to look at some of the background to the safety and risk experiences of children in Corkerhill. This work, which was not costly, was funded through the small grants scheme administered by the trustees of the Nuffield Foundation.

Our contacts in the community helped us recruit the groups in line with guidelines we suggested on selection criteria. To the bemusement of some of our colleagues in the accident-prevention field, we did not get together groups of lone mothers, or groups of people whose children had experienced an accident, or groups living in overcrowded or temporary accommodation. In choosing groups from different housing types, we wanted to understand the role played by different domestic, design and environmental settings in prompting feelings about, actions related to, or anxieties concerning, safety. Materially, we were able to offer the group respondents compensation for their time. As Pearson *et al.* (1993) have shown, far from being a commodity in plentiful supply for those not in paid employment, time is a means of exchange, and very frequently a gift. The groups were recruited with the help of members of the community, and we met in the community 'shop' premises, which are within easy walking distance of every house in Corkerhill. The 'lay' voices met with us on several occasions. Two senior researchers (Helen Roberts and Susan Smith) conducted these interviews, as one way of underlining the importance we placed on these initial soundings. From this work, we were able to build up a picture of the risks and dangers considered salient in the area, and some of the strategies used to reduce risk. This preliminary work is described elsewhere (Roberts *et al.* 1992), and indicated an untapped reservoir of knowledge.

We intended to use this work as the basis for a more ambitious study designed to identify the causes and consequences of child accidents in a high-risk area and to explore the relevance of local knowledge for accident prevention policy. For this, we needed modest funding for around eighteenth months.

Funding

The Economic and Social Research Council (ESRC) declined to fund the research, although it was alpha-rated and therefore 'one of those which the Board wished to support in principle, but for which insufficient funds were available'. One otherwise favourable ('I feel that the sum requested is modest and that the project would probably constitute extremely good "value for money"') and helpful referee's report noted a possible methodological problem concerning 'the disclosure of acts which might put the respondent in an unfavourable light. Respondents . . . may not divulge acts of omission which placed their children in danger. There is a great deal of parental guilt about childhood accidents and near misses. Thus personal accounts and admissions may be edited.'

We *were* collecting data on accidents, but in a context which draws on people's competences. We were interested in how people *prevent* accidents, and our data were being collected on why these strategies – which all households, even 'deficient' ones, practice every day – sometimes fail. Of course, there may well be data which were withheld, although our impression is one of 'over-reporting' by parents (when we compare their reports, for instance, with routinely collected data), rather than under-reporting.

The ESRC currently has under way an initiative on risk and human behaviour. Had we applied for research funds within that initiative, we might have had more luck. But perhaps not. The 'lay voice' in the programme specification is presented as one whose concerns are not necessarily reasonable: 'publicity given to . . . hazards such as salmonella, or nuclear power, has generated public concern over the perceived risks on a scale unsubstantiated statistically or scientifically . . . ' (Economic and Social Research Council, 1993: 2). Risks which are unsubstantiated scientifically may still be risks. An example from Corkerhill is probably replicated all over the country. There is a busy main road on the edge of Corkerhill where a fast dual carriageway narrows to single-lane traffic and a hump-backed bridge. Many parents identified this road as dangerous. 'No' they were told by local experts, 'it is not a blackspot'. In a sense, both parties are right. It *is* a dangerous road, yet there are fewer accidents there than in some other parts of Glasgow – simply because local people avoid crossing it. Although there is a playpark on the far side, it is one of the places identified by parents as somewhere they do not allow children to go. It is too risky to cross, and experience has shown that the pelican crossing is no deterrent to the fast driver. To start with, one parent observed, 'Sometimes these lights are not working . . . . These lights are always breaking down.' In addition, the number of near-misses there has frightened parents into avoidance strategies: 'So many of them [drivers] go through the red lights that it is unbelievable. So if you were a little kid you wouldn't have a chance . . . the adults can hardly watch themselves crossing the road.'

We wanted to produce a study which began with local knowledge and used it to inform policy, not vice versa. The work was finally funded by the Scottish Office Home and Health Department for a period of twelve months. In order to complete the study within this timescale, we had to lose one part of the work which we had intended to do on a child's-eye view of accidents. Thus, although children were central to our research, with the exception of the teenagers we interviewed, they were largely silent subjects.

The second stage: the household survey

For the second part of the study, the household survey, we depended in very large part on our joint work with the community. The survey instrument was developed and refined in close consultation with people in the community and drew on issues raised in the group interviews. The pilots were discussed with members of the community. A television series on child safety, *Play It Safe*, was being filmed at the time our work on the household survey was about to begin, and a community member and one of the researchers were interviewed for the introductory programme. This meant that we were able to send a letter round the community (delivered by community members) reminding people to watch their neighbour on the television at the same time as reminding them of our survey. Walter Morrison and Cathie Rice ensured that notices were put up about the survey in the window of the community shop and lost no opportunity to encourage people to take part. Betty Campbell welcomed and cared for our interviewers, ensuring that the community shop was warm (no mean feat in a Glasgow winter) and that cups of tea and coffee were available.

We had originally planned to train local people as 'lay epidemiologists' to carry out the interviewing. A number of local people already had considerable experience in interviewing for their own surveys. We felt that providing some solid training would be a way of using and developing people's expertise, and leaving at least some people in the community with a potentially marketable skill at the end of the project. This foundered on a number of ethical and financial issues around the provision of short-term, relatively highly paid work for a small number of people in a community suffering very high levels of unemployment. This included the experience of some local people who had taken on short-term jobs only to find that after the jobs came to an end it could take weeks or months to regain all the benefits to which they were entitled. As far as local people were concerned, an over-riding factor was their need for the work to be seen as 'scientific', and this required the use of trained, experienced interviewers. In the event, we used six interviewers with health visitor training, and two without. Most of the interviewers already had considerable experience of interviewing for social research, as they had worked for the Medical Research Council's medical sociology unit in Glasgow. They were given not only professional training for this particular study, but also a day of 'induction' into the community by a local community police officer and Cathie, Walter and Betty, who were our community consultants.

During the course of the study, residents were reminded of interviews by members of the local community, and occasionally a member of the community would accompany one of our interviewers. This would happen if we knew the householder had a hearing problem, or was frail and would be reassured by the presence of a local face.

The third stage: case studies

The third part of our work built on the survey, and comprised case studies of successful and unsuccessful accident prevention strategies. One component of the survey had involved data collection on the epidemiology of accidents in Corkerhill. Data were collected on in-patient admissions and attendances at accident and emergency departments, general practitioner (GP) surgeries and the dentist, following an injury, as well as accidents dealt with without resort to a doctor, nurse or dentist. In addition to those accidents which had resulted in an injury, we collected data on those which did not. The same event (such as sticking a knitting needle into an electric socket) may result in death, serious injury, slight injury or no injury. We therefore collected data on dangerous events not resulting in an injury (on the grounds that they may determine future behaviour) and accidents which had been averted at the last minute, by the child, by the carer or by some other person. From the large number of 'cases' generated, we derived twenty-five accident events for which we conducted lengthy case studies. Although data are often and routinely collected on the sequelae of accidents, that is injuries, very little in the way of systematic data is collected on their antecedents. But it is the antecedents that we need to know more about if we want to prevent accidents. In spite of the sensitivity of the subject, all the parents we approached for case-study data agreed to be interviewed. Indeed, the response rates overall were unusually high, with 92 per cent of households with a child aged 14 or under agreeing to be interviewed.

AT THE END OF THE DAY . . .

At the end of the day the researchers' story is that this piece of work was 'successful'. We had high response rates; we obtained interesting, useful, meaningful data. A book and numerous articles are being written. We have made efforts to disseminate the work in trade and popular journals as well as those scholarly outlets of interest to the Higher Education Funding Council (Roberts 1991; Bryce *et al.* 1992; Smith and Roberts 1991). Papers have been delivered in a variety of settings, involving sometimes the researchers, sometimes people from the community, sometimes both. It is within the spirit of the work that two members of the community, Walter Morrison and Betty Campbell, and not the researchers, attended the World Conference on Injury Prevention organized by the Centers for Disease Control at Atlanta, Georgia.

The details of our findings are published elsewhere (Roberts *et al.* 1995). We believe they show convincingly that the physical environment of Corkerhill puts children at risk, that parents are acutely aware of these risks, and that they take many practical and imaginative steps to keep their children safe. Safety behaviours are more common and valued than risky behaviours, and to a large extent the limits on child safety have more to do with design and adaptability than with knowledge and motivation. In short, parents in Corkerhill have a keen sense of when, where and why their children are in danger. They have developed safety routines which may avert as many as one in five potential accidents, and they have a wealth of cost-effective ideas about ways in which local risks could further be reduced. Local knowledge can, we believe, make a valuable contribution to accident-prevention policy, and what is required to make this happen is not education, but investment in the built and lived environment.

This account of a community-led research programme may make

gaining the trust of a community like Corkerhill seem easy. This is not necessarily the case. As Cathie points out, communities like theirs get tired of 'being researched upon'. An illustration of trust that was built between researchers, interviewers, and the community in Corkerhill can be given by means of a tale that reached us as we were in the middle of fieldwork. At the same time as our interviewers were knocking on doors asking for up to an hour of parents' time, other 'strangers' appeared in Corkerhill wanting people to answer a 'short questionnaire'. These interviewers got little in the way of response from the local residents. They had appeared on residents' doorsteps 'cold', and understandably the residents were wary. Through hearing of this both interviewers and researchers were reminded of the importance of being accepted in a community (in our case through the hard work of the community council) and being trusted.

For the researchers, the study was an enjoyable piece of work, and we are still in contact with some people in the community. While none of us is in the same post she occupied at the time the study started, we all retain an interest in child safety. But at the end of the day we do not live with the problem, or not in such an acute form as the people in Corkerhill. Some changes in safety practices occurred during and after the research. The installation of smoke alarms in Corkerhill coincided with the end of the project (we shall put it no stronger than that). At the time of our household survey 70 per cent of people in Corkerhill did not have a functioning smoke alarm. The slow pace of change sometimes leads us to feel that the most tangible health gain in Corkerhill as a direct result of the research may have been the trip to an injury prevention conference in the USA of two of the residents.

But this may be over-pessimistic. There have been other health gains. Every Sunday, Wednesday and Friday, up to fifty local children join the local 'Dangerwatch' scheme run by Betty Campbell. Rather than being 'talked at' about safety, children are given the much more interesting job of identifying dangers, and asked to keep their eyes open for anything that could cause an accident in their homes, backcourts and streets. A new playgroup, 'The Wee Horrors', was set up. Home-security spyholes in the front door, fire blankets, and doorchains are all on the local agenda, and there is a whole new shopping-list of safety requirements concerning safe play, asbestos removal and traffic calming.

Towards the end of 1993, Glasgow City Council made the decision to invest £970,000 in a central-heating system for Corkerhill. This was probably the result of a number of initiatives. It started with the damp-house inquiry in Corkerhill, then Corkerhill Community Council made representations to the Scottish Office, and then there was evidence from our own research on the risks people perceived as being related to their cold, damp housing. While in traditional accident prevention terms the installation of central heating might seem a long way from getting children to cross roads safely, from the tenants' perspective a warm house is likely to be a safer house for their children.

The experience of working with the project was probably a factor in Cathie Rice getting her job in Safe Levern/Pollock, and many friendships were forged as a result of the research – not just between researchers and the community, but also between interviewers and members of the community. Far from our feeling that human intercourse, networks and social contact invalidate our research, they were vital to it. Between us, we were asked about, or were given advice on, everything from education to filling in forms for the housing department, from bus routes to curtain material. Giving and receiving this kind of advice is the sort of reciprocity that most of us count on in our everyday lives. We feel that it strengthened the data which people were willing to share with us, and the fact that we *listened* to them and *heard* what they said may not be without health-gain potential. The debilitating effects of knowing what is wrong, but not being heard, must be very strong in a community like Corkerhill, and it is a testimony to their resilience that people in Corkerhill continue to work for change.

While people in Corkerhill were partners in the research in more than a superficial sense, it would be disingenuous to suggest that our interests as researchers, and theirs as people wanting to create and maintain a safe community, coincided at every point. There are different interests at stake, and while at one level members of the community may have an intellectual curiosity, as we do, in safety as a social value, their concerns are naturally focused on immediate rather than longer-term strategies for reducing accidents.

What people in Corkerhill need are better playgrounds now, safe electrics now (only one household in five had on/off switches on all their electric sockets); a dry house now (48 per cent of households had a room or rooms unusable because of dampness, poor repair, or heating problems) and thermostats on their hot-water tanks (86 per cent were unable to turn down the temperature in their water tank), to name only some of the problems looking for solutions. The *findings* of research on safety as a social value are unlikely to lead to improvements in these areas, but they are one resource which can be used by an already resourceful community.

The community recognized the need to make alliances with decision-makers, policy-makers and implementers if the project was to be more than parochial in the very strict meaning of the word. As it happens, the work and the community have drawn far more attention from outside the immediate neighbourhood, and even outside Scotland, than they have done locally.

Neither we nor the community are in a position to provide a knitting pattern for safety, but we have collected data which could provide the basis for improving safety at home, at play and in transit at the community level. The combination of the research project and the parents' action group is one we feel may be an effective way of producing local safety data and exploring ways of making communities safer for children.

ACKNOWLEDGEMENTS

Our first acknowledgement is to the people of Corkerhill, who were our co-workers in this study. We are grateful in particular to Betty Campbell and Walter Morrison for their comments on the chapter, and to Wendy Hopkins for her help with word processing.

REFERENCES

Avery, J.G., Vaudin, J.N., Fletcher, J.L., and Watson, J.M. (1990) 'Geographical and social variations in mortality due to childhood accidents in England and Wales 1975–1984', *Public Health* 104: 171–82.

Bryce, C., Roberts, H., and Smith, S.J. (1992) 'It's not all fireguards and safety gates', *THS Health Summary*, April: 7–8.

—— (1993) *Safety as a Social Value: A Community Study of Child Accidents*, Glasgow: Public Health Research Unit, University of Glasgow.

Department of Health (1992) *The Health of the Nation; A Strategy for Health in England*, London: HMSO.

Economic and Social Research Council (1993) *Risk and Human Behaviour Research Programme, Phase I, Programme Specification*, Swindon: Economic and Social Research Council.

Graham, H. (1982) 'Coping, or How mothers are seen and not heard', in Friedman, S., and Sarah, E., eds, *On the Problems of Men*, London: The Women's Press.

Martin, C.J., Platt, S.D., and Hunt, S.M. (1987) 'Housing conditions and ill health', *British Medical Journal* 294: 1125–7.

Morrison, W., Rice, C., Roberts, H., and Svanström, L. (1992) *Corkerhill, Glasgow: Application to Become a Member of the Safe Community Network*, Paper no. 275, Sundbyberg: Karolinska Institute, Department of Social Medicine.

Oxford, E. (1993) 'The village that is sick of living without a future', *Independent on Sunday* 15 August: 5.

Pearson, M., Dawson, F., Moore, H., and Spencer, S., (1993) 'Health on borrowed time: prioritising and meeting needs in low income households', *Health and Social Care 1*: 45–54.

Pless, I.B., Peckham, C.S., and Power, C. (1989) 'Predicting traffic injuries in childhood – a cohort analysis', *Journal of Paediatrics* 115, 6: 932–8.

Roberts, H., (1991) 'Accident prevention: a community approach', *Health Visitor* 64, 7: 219–21.

Roberts, H., Smith, S.J., and Lloyd, M. (1992) 'Safety as a social value: a community approach,' in Scott, S., Williams, G., Platt, S., and Thomas, H., eds, *Private Risks and Public Dangers*, Basingstoke: Avebury Press.

Roberts, H., Smith, S.J., and Bryce, C. (1993) 'Prevention is better . . . ', *Sociology of Health and Illness*', 15, 4: 447–63.

Roberts, H., Smira, S.J., and Bryd, C. (1995) *Children at Risk*, Milton Keynes: Open University Press.

Smith, S.J., and Roberts, H. (1991) 'Accident prevention and local knowledge,' *THS Health Summary*, October: 5–6.

Stone, D., with Roberts, H. (1992) *Housing and Health* (training video for general practitioners), Glasgow: Public Health Research Unit, University of Glasgow.

Towner, E., Dowswell, T., and Jarvis, S. (1993) *Reducing Childhood Accidents: The Effectiveness of Health Promotion Interventions: A Literature Review*, London: Health Education Authority.

Wadsworth, I., Burnell, I., Taylor, J., and Butler, W. (1983) 'Family type and accidents in pre-school children', *Journal of Epidemiology and Community Health* 37: 100–4.

Worfwel, E., and de Geus, G.H. (1993) 'Prevention of home related injuries of pre-school children: safety measures taken by mothers', *Health Education Research* 8, 2: 217–31.

Chapter 8

Discounted knowledge

Local experience, environmental pollution and health

Peter Phillimore and Suzanne Moffatt

INTRODUCTION

The last decade has seen a resurgence of public concern about the physical environment, which has taken two main forms. Most publicized has been concern with the global consequences of our collective use of the planet. But comparable concern has been aroused, on a quite different geographical scale, about particular sources of pollution and the local populations living nearby. This chapter is about the latter, and about the social and political context in which such concerns are expressed and contested. We shall draw on two case studies from major urban centres in north-east England to explore some of the methodological issues which arise from trying to take local understandings seriously in research of an epidemiological nature.

Where people have voiced anxieties about the effects upon their health of pollution from an individual factory or industrial process, a common official response in the initial stages of what often turns out to be a long-running issue has been to dismiss public fears as unnecessary and exaggerated. In our experience, this is often accompanied by the rider that concern about personal smoking habits would be more rational and effective – an interesting juxtaposition of air-pollution concerns about which we shall have more to say later. Another dismissive response is to minimize public concerns by suggesting that only a minority worry about pollution. With an implied claim to be portraying the views of the majority, the argument goes that employment security and local crime are greater local preoccupations than pollution. These official responses have the effect of foreclosing debate: local voices may not be stifled but they are largely ignored. Since these voices are more often than not those of working-class people living in neighbourhoods where economic hardship is common, questions of power and inequality are necessarily involved.

Nevertheless, over the last few years a gradual reassessment of the possible impact of air pollution on health has been occurring. This comes after a long period of dormancy, in the wake of the large reductions in smoke and sulphur dioxide levels achieved through progressive implementation of the Clean Air Act and the introduction of smokeless zones in most cities. A recent editorial in *The Lancet*, under the title 'Environmental pollution: it kills trees, but does it kill people?' (1992: 821), is one indication of this shift. The issues here are not only epidemiological or toxicological. The way that concerns about health and environmental pollution take shape in the public arena – the timing, the interests and coalitions involved, the problems identified – reflects processes of interest to sociologists and anthropologists. One recurrent topic in local environmental controversies is the weight that should be given to the knowledge and experience of those who either claim that their health has been affected or are worried about a possible effect. How seriously are such claims and concerns to be taken? And what are the implications for methodology of taking these claims seriously?

Let us suppose that people in a community express unease about the effects on their health of environmental pollution from a nearby industry, and a subsequent health survey shows raised levels of self-reported respiratory symptoms. On what grounds do we conclude either that the evidence confirms local public unease, or alternatively that the population concerned is so predisposed towards the possibility of a health effect that the apparent evidence must be discounted as 'reporting bias'? The question is far from academic, for a common undercurrent when a local issue emerges is that people living close to the pollution source in question face an uphill struggle to have their concerns taken seriously. Around the Monkton coking works, in Hebburn on the south side of the River Tyne, these concerns were often expressed in remarks like the following by a 52-year-old woman living in the vicinity of the works. The comment is of interest precisely because of the way in which it echoes the question posed by *The Lancet*: 'I am a keen gardener. In the last 20 years, 3 apple trees have died . . . apples were black, sticky and attracted flies. You couldn't open your windows for the sulphur smells in summer. If the plants and trees were dying, the air pollution couldn't have done me much good.'

This chapter is primarily about the role of local knowledge and belief in guiding epidemiological attempts to explore links between industrial air pollution and the health of people living nearby. In other words, it is about themes that have been associated with the concept of 'popular epidemiology' (Brown 1992; Paigen 1982), and looks at some of the difficulties that arise with environmental controversies in interpreting data on the elusive phenomenon of illness or morbidity. To set the scene, however, we will first outline the background to the two studies which give rise to this discussion, giving particular emphasis to the contexts in which the research takes place, the interested parties, and the relationships between researchers and researched.

BACKGROUND TO STUDIES IN TYNESIDE AND TEESSIDE

In the first case to be described, in Tyneside, popular concern played a leading role in bringing about an empirical study: the research was a response to a long local debate. In the second case, in Teesside, research played more of an initiating role in the debate that developed through the later 1980s.

The coking works at Monkton, in the Hebburn area of South Tyneside, started operating in 1937, but it was in the 1980s that it became a source of local controversy, which continued until its sudden closure late in 1990. Concern can be traced back to the 1950s, when the post-war wave of slum clearance in Hebburn and Jarrow led to a series of new housing estates – predominantly council-owned – being built close to what had formerly been the relatively isolated site of the coking works. When the Lukes Lane council estate was started in the late 1960s the National Coal Board itself questioned the desirability of siting housing half a mile downwind of coking production. That historical fact was something local residents generally acknowledged, even when uneasy about the effects of atmospheric pollutants from the works: 'The coke ovens were there first, not houses, so the council in my opinion were responsible and shouldn't have built the houses so close.'

By the end of the 1970s a widespread expectation among residents seems to have been that the Monkton site was in the later stages of its life. But in 1980 a return to twin-battery production (sixty-six coke ovens instead of thirty-three), after the works had operated with only one battery for most of its history, overturned such assumptions, and led directly to the creation of a residents' action group in Hebburn, initially to campaign about the levels of pollution from the works.

Through the 1980s local concerns were voiced with growing frequency, several factors playing a part. Hebburn and Jarrow had been smokeless zones since 1968, and living in an area free of domestic smoke but alongside a plant burning coal to make coke increasingly came to be seen as an unacceptable anomaly. The decline of heavy industry in the area might have made the preservation of jobs at the coking works a local priority sufficient to counteract environmental concerns. But not only did the decline in heavy industry mark out the Monkton works as one of the few remaining sources of pollution; it equally highlighted the fact that coke production had never formed part of the identity of the area in the way that ship-building and coal-mining had done. The Monkton works could not therefore call on the same local loyalty that pits or shipyards evoked. If this was so before the national miners' strike of 1984–5, it became even more the case afterwards, for redundancies and redeployment from other sites in the north-east ensured that from 1986 onwards less than 5 per cent of the workforce of about two hundred lived in the vicinity of the works.

The period 1986–90 saw local concern start to focus more on health issues: partly, we suspect, spurred on by the fact that closure during the miners' strike and for several months afterwards (twenty-one months in all) had provided residents with an unexpected natural experiment, in which they assessed for themselves the changes to their immediate environment and their health brought about by the stopping and then the restarting of coking operations. Several developments helped to give momentum to the campaign by local activists. A planning application by the company in 1987 to use waste gas from the coking process, at the time being flared, to generate electricity, was subject to two public inquiries, the first in 1987, with a second, reopened inquiry in 1990. These provided a public forum in which health issues received unprecedented local attention, the residents' action group financing the presentation of its own case both times. Between these two occasions the residents' group also pressed its case by conducting its own self-designed survey of residents' health in the areas closest to the coking works. The paradox of this initiative in self-help research was that while its findings were discounted ('unscientific') it proved an effective political instrument in persuading local and health authorities to give greater recognition to such manifest local unease. The decision in 1989 by South Tyneside Metropolitan Borough Council (MBC) to fund research into the possible health effects of air pollution from the Monkton coking works was thus the culmination of years of increasingly vocal concern by local residents, in a context of changing perceptions about environmental health questions.

Before the research had been under way a year, however, coking operations at Monkton finally ceased. Not surprisingly, this sudden closure forced abrupt changes in research plans, but it was not without advantages, providing an opportunity for some 'before and after' comparisons of both environmental data and evidence on health (Bhopal *et al.* 1992).

In Teesside, home of the largest concentration of steel and petro-chemical industries in Britain, the context in which the research emerged is somewhat different. There, possible problems associated with air pollution stand out less starkly alongside acute problems of unemployment, consequent poverty, and housing problems in some areas (Beynon *et al.* 1989; Centre for Environmental Studies 1985; Hudson 1990; Sadler 1990).[1] Until the large-scale redundancies of the 1980s, which gave Cleveland the highest unemployment rate in mainland Britain, the local estates were heavily dependent on employment in steel and chemicals; and despite massive contraction these industries are still seen as the essential base for the long-term viability of the area's economy.

Against this background, research into health and environmental pollution in Teesside developed less from the concerns of local residents and more from a combination of general practitioners' (GPs') concerns about the health problems of their patients, coupled with research studies which showed that many of the poorer areas of Teesside experienced exceptional levels of premature mortality (Townsend *et al.* 1988; Phillimore and Morris 1991; Phillimore 1993). Whereas in South Tyneside our study started without any prior research to support residents' claims about a health effect from industrial pollution, in Teesside recent research had been instrumental in establishing that a health problem existed which required further scrutiny.

A feature common to both places, however, has been recent interest in testing legal claims through the courts against particular companies for damage to health arising from living close to polluting operations. The possibility of making legal claims based on residential, instead of occupational, exposure to toxic substances is a new development in Britain, and much of the initiative here has come from law firms with special interests in this field. But potential claimants have been ready to come forward, and the eventual outcomes of Monkton and Teesside cases are likely to set precedents which will be of national importance. In the context of the Monkton research, the possibility of litigation only emerged towards the end of the study and had no bearing on its conduct. But in Teesside, the likelihood of future litigation has introduced another set of participants into the story at an early stage, and already colours any dialogue between the main Teesside industries and researchers, for claims are unlikely to be pursued in the courts until the findings of the present study are available.[2]

There was one further rationale for research in Teesside, which had little to do with local pressures and concerns. Teesside in this context simply provided a peculiarly appropriate setting to try to answer questions of wider interest about the impact of industrial air pollution on the health of local populations. One proposition underlying the present research programme may be expressed in these terms. If air pollution from industrial sources remains a hazard to human health at non-occupational levels of exposure anywhere in Britain, then the scale of steel and petro-chemical industries and the proximity of residential neighbourhoods in Teesside mean that significant effects are more likely to be demonstrable there than elsewhere. Should such significant effects not be found in Teesside, then the likelihood must be that industrial air pollution is not a serious contributor to public ill-health elsewhere in Britain. Moreover, the proximity of populations already known to experience severe material hardship enables us to explore the cumulative effects of air pollution in conjunction with other forms of poverty. In part, this work also arose, therefore, out of an extension into the environmental field of long-standing debates about health and poverty.

Despite the different ways in which research on air pollution emerged on local policy agendas in the two settings, it would be mistaken to conclude that environmental concerns have been dormant in Teesside. Public preoccupation in recent years has centred around new and planned developments (a toxic waste incinerator on the north side of the River Tees, and a new power station on the south side) rather than around existing operations. In the public debate these new developments have generated, a recurring theme has been the pollution burden Teesside already carries, and hostility to its enlargement. Concerns exist, therefore, but possible threats posed to health have generally been less tangible, and accorded a lower priority, than the daily economic pressures and material hardships of a decade of exceptionally high unemployment. A further difference between the two areas lies in the geographical scale involved. In contrast to the relatively compact boundaries of the Monkton controversy, potentially affected populations in Teesside are dispersed across a wide area. Inevitably, this makes it impossible to speak of a local community such as surrounds the Monkton coking works, for in Teesside there are several such areas. While the main illustration we use here is drawn from Monkton, where research has been completed, our understanding of the issues has developed just as much through our experience of research in Teesside.

TAKING LOCAL VOICES SERIOUSLY

Studies into possible health effects of pollution from industry might be expected to involve the people defined as being at risk, namely those living alongside these industries. Yet a thread running through the Monkton case, and a persistent undercurrent both in Teesside and elsewhere (Irwin and Wynne forthcoming), is that the issues are for scientific experts alone to evaluate. The subjects of study are thus human guinea-pigs, whose views of their experience are at best beside the point and at worst an obstacle to proper scientific assessment of the facts. Taking local concerns seriously in this context means challenging such a standpoint on two complementary levels. One is to re-assess the empirical evaluation of health, to take account of local experience in the ways that episodes of illness and pollution are actually measured. A second is to step back from questions of measurement and quantitative assessment, to explore the extent to which different 'ways of knowing' (Brown 1992) about the environment and its impact on human health shape disputes between residents who see themselves as being on the receiving end of pollution, and public authorities and professional advisers who base their assessments and policy responses on 'official' forms of knowledge (see also Irwin and Wynne forthcoming). These two levels reflect the duality of processes which are both socially caused and socially constructed. Scott and Williams emphasize the second of these when they write:

> What is of central concern to sociologists, in contrast perhaps to their colleagues in public health, is not the evaluation of risk and danger in any absolute sense, but rather our shifting perceptions of risk and changing patterns of risk management.
>
> (Scott and Williams 1992: 3)

However, questions of empirical measurement are likely to have great importance for local communities confronting public authorities in environmental disputes. The possibility of bringing about changes in policy that will have an impact on the immediate environment rests on the authority of the empirical evidence that can be marshalled in support of any contention about actual or potential adverse effects on health or daily lives. In short, the public priority is generally to know whether scientific findings identify harmful effects on health.

In the planning stages of the Monkton study, a recurring theme in descriptions by local residents of how coking pollution affected them was that short periods of severe pollution, perhaps lasting no more than a few minutes, could trigger off bouts of respiratory illness that could linger on for several days. The emphasis in these accounts tended to be on the way that pollution incidents exacerbated chronic respiratory conditions. Particularly in the housing estates closest to the coking works, such localized pollution peaks were typically associated with the regular sequence of 'pushing' the coke from the ovens every twenty minutes or so, when meteorological conditions could readily combine with incomplete carbonization to produce intense fumes in a fairly small area. Such conditions were quite distinct from the continuous emissions of waste gases through the stack, which tended to be spread more widely but in more diluted form. While temperature-inversion conditions are well known as danger signs for the trapping of polluted air, often over quite a large area, the gist of our informants' experience was that blustery wind conditions could also be a significant but localized problem, for when the coke ovens were pushed swirling clouds of gas and smoke would sweep over some houses but not others. Yet pollution such as this, emitted close to ground level, is much harder to monitor and quantify than emissions from chimneys, which are subject to greater regulation. Scientific predictions about exposure are therefore based almost exclusively upon stack emissions, not those fugitive and other emissions occurring close to ground level.

Here, then, was a description of one way that pollution from the coking works was observed to take a toll on health. Speculation was widespread about hidden health effects with a latency period of years, notably in relation to cancers; but the difference in this case was that observation and personal experience linked cause and effect together directly because there was no time-lag to speak of between the two to obscure a link. Yet, however significant as personal experience, such observations also provided a cue for empirical investigation. Indeed, such investigation was essential if findings were to carry weight with bureaucracies and policy-makers. We approached this question by using air-pollution data from three monitoring sites set up by South Tyneside MBC from 1986 onwards to monitor smoke and sulphur dioxide levels around the coking works. Pollution data averaged by week or month were insufficiently sensitive for our purpose. Disaggregated data were essential to enable us to construct mean daily levels of pollution to match with daily data on consultations with a GP. This level of temporal disaggregation proved sufficiently sensitive to reveal a strong association between sulphur dioxide levels and the rate of consultation for respiratory problems on the same day. In view of that pattern, any further disaggregation – for instance to three-hourly intervals – seemed redundant, though in theory that would have been the next step towards assessment of local claims. The empirical evidence has been summarized elsewhere and will not be reviewed here (Bhopal *et al.* 1994). It is sufficient to say that standard epidemiological methods of analysis were used before we concluded that the association between sulphur dioxide levels and consultations for respiratory complaints was largely attributable to air pollution from the coking works. These methods included: comparison with a control population elsewhere in the borough of South Tyneside; examination of differences between patterns for respiratory and all other problems; scrutiny of patterns before and after coking operations finally ceased; separation of the effects of air temperature from those of pollution; and a check on alternative pollution sources.

While acknowledging that consultations with a GP provide only an indirect reflection of morbidity or illness patterns, on the face of it this evidence would seem to lend support to claims by residents that pollution from the coking works had harmed their health. It also lends weight to arguments in favour of recognizing, and not ignoring, the insights which come from direct familiarity with a local environment. Brown expresses these well,[3] and reverses the usual emphasis on the shortcomings of popular scientific understanding, stressing instead the limitations of the data available to scientists:

> Many people who live at risk of toxic hazards have access to data otherwise inaccessible to scientists. Their experiential knowledge usually precedes official and scientific awareness, largely because it is so tangible. Knowledge of toxic hazards in communities and workplaces in the last two decades has often stemmed from lay observation.
>
> (Brown 1992: 270)

Nevertheless, findings such as those mentioned above are commonly contested by epidemiologists, and 'reporting bias' is the main explanation given for such scepticism. In essence, the critique goes that the strength of pre-existing local concern about possible health effects of pollution is so great as to predispose a population to think that their health is being harmed. For example, the possibility cannot be ruled out that people in exposed neighbourhoods will anticipate health problems on days when they are aware that pollution is worse than usual, and go to see a doctor. The fact that the Monkton study found the association to be strongest between pollution level and consultation with a doctor on the same day may reinforce doubts about the interpretation of these linked observations, for it might plausibly be argued that a time-lag between pollution incident and consultation would be more realistic. But the issue goes beyond dispute over one specific set of empirical findings or another, raising general questions to do with the interpretation of evidence where public controversy predates and surrounds scientific inquiry.

The standard argument in epidemiological studies is that human awareness of a health issue introduces a source of potential bias in any assessment of 'health behaviour' which is difficult to control for, compromising the use of self-reports of health states, and such actions as visiting a doctor. The influence of the double-blind trial and case-control methodology looms large here, with the premise that scientific knowledge is produced by screening off the intrusions of life outside the experiment. Prior familiarity with an issue is not seen as a source of insight and the product of experience, but is categorized as 'sensitization', the social equivalent of an allergic response. Given that it may well be impossible to demonstrate that epidemiological findings on any group of people known to be aware of a health issue are unbiased by their prior sensitization to this issue, it means that relatively subtle health effects may never adequately be recognized. *The Lancet* editorial, quoted previously, concluded by stating (1992: 822): 'From published evidence, environmental pollution is unlikely to result in gross excess mortality . . . . Effects should be sought at more subtle levels of health damage – for example, reproductive and developmental outcomes *and morbidity*' (our emphasis). Yet what kind of evidence of morbidity would not be vulnerable to the charge of the sceptical epidemiologist that it was simply an artefact?

For those who do not consider direct familiarity and experience should be underestimated, however, the main problem with this perspective is the assumption that the awareness, or knowledge, of those studied is an obstacle to researchers' knowledge. Indeed, if people's awareness poses problems, one could equally argue that so too would being totally unaware, inasmuch as people need to understand what they are being asked about sufficiently to provide intelligible answers in research. That our subjects of study have prior 'awareness' of the topics we are looking at is a precondition for our knowledge as researchers. One consequence of seeing popular awareness as an obstacle to scientific understanding of behaviour is that it implicitly assumes that people's thoughts distort their 'natural' behaviour. A notion such as 'over-visiting' the doctor (a relevant topic in a discussion of reporting bias) could only come from such a tradition of thinking about human behaviour. The underlying assumption present in such instances is of an implicit dichotomy between 'real' need and 'artificial' (that is to say, culturally created) need. Yet as Blaxter among others has shown (1985, 1990), distinguishing a biological bedrock against which the cultural enactment of illness may be judged is beset by pitfalls in practice and flawed as an idea.

The complex relationship between the social and the biological is also apparent if we go back to the two complementary approaches to lay knowledge and subjective experience that we mentioned earlier. Lay beliefs offer on the one hand an insight into a cultural perspective on the world, and on the other a possible guide to aetiology, a source of hypotheses about causal pathways to disease which may be translated into the idiom of scientific research design. Both of these frameworks for understanding pose characteristic dilemmas. From an aetiological perspective, the paradox of popular epidemiology is this: if local knowledge is not used to enhance the sensitivity of studies measuring the health impact of environmental pollution, then possible effects may go undetected. Such circumstances simply reinforce the epidemiological tendency towards false negative rather than false positive reports noted by various commentators (Brown 1992; Paigen 1982). On the other hand, if local knowledge is used it may lead critics to dispute positive findings on the grounds that the subjects of the study were sensitized to the issue beforehand, thus predisposing them towards the possibility of reporting health effects. There is no straightforward resolution of this problem.

From a social-construction perspective, justice can be done to the subtlety and distinctiveness of popular understandings of environmental hazards, toxic effects and health impacts in different localities. In theory, the authenticity and strength of the account does not depend on validating interpretations by reference to bio-medical data. Yet in practice resort may be made to bio-medical criteria, as a kind of gold standard against which to judge how well founded local knowledge proves to be, and to underscore the argument for taking it seriously. Thus, Brown's fascinating analysis (1992) of the controversy surrounding the explanation for an apparent cluster of childhood leukaemia cases at Woburn, Massachusetts, rests on the assumption that there is a biological foundation on which the social 'story' of the dispute can be built. Likewise, Scott (1988) concludes his account of the different languages of medical, scientific and legal scrutiny of possible cases arising from exposure to the herbicide Agent Orange, by reference to likely biological confirmation of the effects of exposure, as raised levels of certain cancers started to appear.

If the dilemma for aetiological use of lay knowledge is that biological effects can never wholly be distinguished from the social discourse in which they emerge as potential data, the dilemma for a constructionist reading is that recourse to biological evidence is an almost inevitable consequence of attempting to demonstrate the wider legitimacy, in a political and social arena, of local claims.[4]

THE POLITICS OF EXCLUSION

We have to remember also that the views and insights of some groups are more readily discounted than those of others. Particularly in environmental controversies where a working-class community finds itself at odds with a major industrial concern, there are likely to be strong political–economic pressures that make it easier to ignore local voices raised in concern (Crenson 1971). As Becker (1967) observed many years ago, a 'hierarchy of credibility' ensures that the unwanted views of certain sections of the population can effectively be discounted. Environmental debates and disputes do not take place in a political vacuum, and where these involve industry, local government and a resident population the political context is potentially a charged one (Hudson 1990). Historically, there have existed strong political pressures inhibiting both scrutiny of air pollution and the possible consequences for public health in towns with a long-lasting reliance on particular heavy industries. Crenson's comparative (1971) study of city-level politics in the steel-making centres of Gary and East Chicago is highly instructive in this context. His examination of the way that air-pollution issues were tentatively addressed in one town and effectively kept out of the political arena in the other, in the years after the Second World War, illuminates how strongly influential industrial–economic interests can determine local and regional political agendas.

Taking seriously the views of the subjects of study is in itself liable to provoke unease among other interested parties – most obviously the industries themselves, but also sometimes local and health authorities, as Paigen (1982) shows. There is a dilemma here. From the research point of view, to investigate thoroughly the possibility of air pollution either triggering episodes of acute respiratory illness or contributing to the onset of chronic conditions probably requires a combination of methods. The more intensive the study, we would argue, the greater the chance of reaching a conclusion that does not leave open the possibility that the methods chosen were simply insufficiently sensitive. At the same time, the development of sufficiently sensitive methods is unlikely to take place unless researchers and others see that there is a case to answer. But to critics, suggesting that there is a case to answer is tantamount to making a false charge, implying a predisposition on the part of the researchers to be biased against the industry under scrutiny.

Although it concerns water-borne, not air-borne pollution, few cases in this context are as instructive as the Love Canal saga (Levine 1982; Paigen 1982). Love Canal, in New York State, was the site of post-Second World War housing which became contaminated when highly toxic chemical waste legally disposed of in an abandoned canal by the Hooker Electrochemical Corporation started to leach into homes and a school playground, raising serious local alarm by the mid-1970s. The communities' concerns about the risks to health received contradictory and ambiguous responses from the relevant authorities, which were compounded by ferocious disputes between scientists and regulatory authorities. One of the scientists on the receiving end of the displeasure of Health Department officials and influential medical scientists concluded that 'the Love Canal controversy was predominantly political in nature, and it raised a series of questions that had more to do with values than science' (Paigen 1982: 29). As the account of a biological scientist, this article by Paigen is particularly interesting on the recognition of the values that underpin scientific research assumptions and design. Some of these points are brought out in a section headed 'The failure to resolve any controversy may be advantageous to one side', where Paigen observes:

> The advantages to delay were graphically brought home to me in a conversation I had with a Health Department epidemiologist concerning the data on adverse pregnancy outcomes at Love Canal. We both agreed that we should take the conservative approach only to find that in every case we disagreed on what the conservative approach was. To him 'conservative' meant that we must be very cautious about concluding that Love Canal was an unsafe place to live. The evidence had to be compelling because substantial financial resources were needed to correct the problem. To me 'conservative' meant that we must be very cautious about concluding that Love Canal was a safe place to live. The evidence had to be compelling because the public health consequences of an error were considerable. And so we disagreed about specific detail after specific detail.
>
> (Paigen 1982: 32)

ALTERNATIVE MEANINGS OF RISK

Much of the conflict in cases like this revolves around the nature and extent of any risk to health. Too often, scientists, local authorities and the industries concerned see complaints and anxieties voiced by the public as out of proportion to the risk posed, or even irrational and anti-scientific. These authorities have their own ideas about 'real' risks, based largely on the ways that individuals behave, denoted in the concept of 'risky behaviour' (British Medical Association 1990). The retort from local communities caught up in an environmental health controversy is of official and expert unconcern. Both sides speak the language of 'risk', but the languages are fundamentally different (see Dake 1992; Douglas 1985). On the one side, risk is a technical term and risk assessment a highly technical matter, to be 'carried out' by experts and then expressed in quantifiable probabilities. On the other side, risk is part of the currency of everyday life, a concept rooted in daily experience and assessed by reference to experience. The one counts, the other does not (see Hayes 1992).[5] Yet the evidence from studies such as that at Monkton is that people weigh up carefully the manifold influences upon their health. They compare their own and their family's health at different periods: before coming to live near the coking works and afterwards, for instance; or the period of closure of the works during the miners' strike with the periods either side; or the interlude away from home provided by going on holiday. They draw on their knowledge of the health of friends or neighbours. And they witness the way that pollution behaves under different weather conditions and by night and day. Taken in the round, they reach a judgement about risk that is informed by as many different variables as make up scientific assessments of risk. The following remarks by residents living close to the coking works illustrate concern about risk based on observation and experience:

> 'I have always believed that the cokeworks were to blame for all my sinus problems as I never had any symptoms before I exchanged houses to my present address. I lived at my previous home for seven years without any sinus problems.'
>
> (Woman, aged 42)

> 'Although I have no noticeable chest or health problems now, after living here 12 years, the unknown factor is the long-term effects of dust on lungs and when or if they show up in 10–20 years' time.'
>
> (Man, aged 39)

An essential feature of such personal judgements is that they are grounded in a local context, and are specific to that context, as Irwin has argued (Irwin and Wynne forthcoming). Using a case study in Manchester, he shows how, in an area associated for many years with one particular industry, residents were far from apathetic or unconcerned, but combined scepticism about information provided by the industry itself or scientific-review bodies with resigned recognition that alternatives to the *status quo* were few.

CONCLUSION

That air pollution from industry can cause severe ill-health and death can hardly be gainsaid. The sulphurous smogs of past decades caused excess deaths in the rich countries of the world, and industries at that time contributed significantly to total pollution (as continues to be the case in poorer countries, including those of Eastern Europe). The disasters of Bhopal and Seveso also provide well-known instances of the possible dangers in the circumstances posed by major accidents.

Nevertheless, several factors have combined to inhibit conclusions about the current role of routinely produced air pollution in contributing to variations in ill-health between cities, or neighbourhoods within cities. It has proved extremely difficult to design studies which can disentangle the effects of air pollution under the operational conditions prevailing today in Western Europe or North America, where pollution is no longer at a level to create short-term fluctuations in mortality (Lippmann and Lioy 1985). Routine emissions may overall be a fraction of their former level; but in particular places short and often localized periods of relatively high exposure continue to occur, and we are a long way from monitoring the range of pollutants released into the air. The problem is accentuated when we consider historical changes, and try to encompass the conditions experienced through the life-course by those who are now in middle age or elderly. As Scott noted in his study of the Agent Orange controversy, with any latent disorders the time-lag between exposure and consequence strains methodologies 'to the point where it is difficult to establish evidence' (1988: 156). When we acknowledge also that people living in more exposed neighbourhoods are likely to have problems of pollution compounded by damp housing, occupational exposure to pollutants, and smoking, these methodological problems are amplified still further. Studies of the steel-foundry towns of Armadale and Bathgate in Scotland by Lloyd and colleagues (Lloyd 1978; Lloyd *et al.* 1985a, 1985b), which indicated raised lung-cancer incidence (as well as distorted sex ratios at birth) in the 1960s and 1970s, stand out as unusual examples of localized effects attributable to industrial pollution.

These well-known methodological problems have provided obstacles to the development of research to clarify the role of air pollution. Yet this is only half the story. The other side of it has to do with the ways that the problem of air pollution and health has been socially and politically constructed, particularly where the impact of pollution from industry is at issue. For not only are studies of industrial air pollution difficult to design; they are also liable to be politically contentious. One consequence of the methodological complexity alluded to has been to protect industries of a polluting kind from close scrutiny. This insulation has allowed industries to maintain confidently that their emissions have no effect, in the knowledge that any conclusions would be hard to reach, and the claims of affected populations, based on experience, easily deflected. On the other hand, by comparison with even a decade ago, there are signs that the situation is changing. Local authorities struggling to attract new investment, particularly in high-tech sectors, find themselves today at an increasing disadvantage if they cannot guarantee environmental standards that would not have been expected in years gone by (Hudson 1990). Such new economic pressures are likely in the long run to sustain greater pressure on those industries which are the major contributors to air pollution than local community or resident groups could ever achieve.

To the extent that the influence of air pollution is examined, moreover, it echoes some of the main features of more general debates about the causes of health variations within the population. Contrasting emphases on the individual and the behavioural – the realm of personal 'lifestyle' – or the structural and societal have their unacknowledged counterparts in air-pollution epidemiology.

Smoking habits – the ultimate in personalized air pollution – and emissions from industrial plants – the epitome of externally imposed air pollution – neatly exhibit the two ends of the spectrum. Traffic-exhaust fumes, and indoor pollution from domestic fuel or even home furnishings and clothing fall somewhere between these two extremes, although there is a tendency to treat all of these as closer to the 'lifestyle' than the structural end of the pollution spectrum. To the extent that individual exposure entails a more-or-less unique combination of these pollutants, it is not surprising that consideration of the effects of external air pollution invariably takes personal smoking habits into account also. But from there it has proved a short step to the discounting of external sources in the case of individuals who smoke. As we mentioned at the start of this chapter, smokers who express concern about air pollution are seen to exemplify an almost irrational concern with a minor and remote problem at the expense of the major and immediate one over which they have personal control. Thus is the ideology of health as an individual achievement brought into air-pollution risk assessment. To put the point differently, here is another instance of the way in which private risks always receive priority over public dangers (Scott *et al.* 1992).

There seems little doubt that the rising tide of environmental pre-occupation will lead to a growing number of epidemiological studies being undertaken against a background of public concern. In this chapter we have explored some of the challenges to received epidemiological ideas posed by public interest in the issues under investigation, and the wider context within which such studies take place. On the one hand, the days of a public who passively have research 'done' on them are disappearing; at the same time, it remains all too easy to discount the voices of those being studied, especially where the issue under scrutiny is – like air pollution – seen as too technical a matter for non-experts to participate in.

Yet one of the main implications of this chapter is that, whatever the methodological challenges involved, the voices of those living in local communities most at risk from possible environmental hazards must be heard. This basic lesson applies both to the range of public authorities which are likely to be the first to respond to local concerns, and to researchers who may come into the picture at a later stage. Assumptions about public misunderstanding, ignorance or hysteria in relation to environmental issues simply fan the flames of controversy, and caricature the insights and understanding people bring to the circumstances in which they find themselves. Instead, as several writers have argued (Brown 1992; Hance *et al.* 1989; Nash and Kirsch 1986), public authorities and research teams need to recognize that the community may very well have expert knowledge about possible routes of exposure, based on long and direct familiarity. This knowledge needs to be respected and sought, so that its implications can be studied thoroughly. In the wake of the infamous Love Canal saga, some of these lessons are being learned in the USA. Researchers involved in the US Environmental Communication Research Program, having examined a number of disputes, recommended 'paying [as much] attention to the community's perception of the risk and to the community's concerns, as to scientific variables' (Hance *et al.* 1989: 114).

NOTES

1 One difference between South Tyneside and Teesside is the amount of recent social science literature on the two places. While there has been a steady stream of publications on Teesside over the last decade or so, little has been written on South Tyneside.

2 The importance of the interplay between scientific findings and legal judgements in the USA has been noted recently by Brown (1992: 279): 'Legal definitions of causality, developed in an expanding toxic tort repertoire, are initially determined by judicial interpretation of scientific testimony. Once constructed, they can take on a life of their own.' See also Scott 1988: 156–8.

3 A similar point is made by Nash and Kirsch in quoting a local figure in a dispute involving contamination by polychlorinated biphenyls in Pittsfield, Massachusetts (1986: 134): 'This is the area we grew up in and we know the problem, better than management. They've only been here a short period of time. I'm sure they meant no harm; they've been cooperative, but nonethe-less, we have the problem.'

4 The discussion between Bryan Turner and Richard Fardon (in Turner 1992: especially pp. 252–6) sets these questions within the broader context of social theory.

5 De Waal's (1989) discussion of alternative understandings of 'famine' – the one technical and quantitative, the other experience-based – in his ethnography of Darfur, in Sudan, provides an apposite parallel to the contrasting notions of risk being explored here.

ACKNOWLEDGEMENTS

The research on which this essay draws has been conducted with Raj Bhopal, Chris Dunn, Chris Foy, and Jacqui Tate. Their role is acknowledged gratefully. We are also indebted to Raj Bhopal, Chris Dunn, Erica Haimes, Jennie Popay and Gareth Williams for constructive criticism of earlier drafts.

REFERENCES

Becker, H. (1967) 'Whose side are we on?', *Social Problems* 14: 239–47.

Beynon, H., Hudson, R., Lewis, J., Sadler, D., and Townsend, A. (1989) '"It's all falling apart here": coming to terms with the future in Teesside', in Cooke, P., ed., *Localities: The changing face of urban Britain*, London: Unwin Hyman.

Bhopal, R., Moffatt, S., Phillimore, P., and Foy, C. (1992) *The Impact of an Industry on the Health of a Community: The Monkton Coking Works Study*, A report to South Tyneside MBC, Newcastle upon Tyne: University of Newcastle upon Tyne.

Bhopal, R., Phillimore, P., Moffatt, S., and Foy, C. (1994) 'Is living near a coking works harmful to health?', *Journal of Epidemiology and Community Health*, 48, 3.

Blaxter, M. (1985) 'Self-definition of health status and consulting rates in primary care', *Quarterly Journal of Social Affairs* 1, 2: 131–71.
—— (1990) *Health and Lifestyles*, London: Tavistock/Routledge.
British Medical Association (1990) *The BMA Guide to Living with Risk*, London: Penguin Books.
Brown, P. (1992) 'Popular epidemiology and toxic waste contamination: lay and professional ways of knowing', *Journal of Health and Social Behaviour* 33: 267–81.
Centre for Environmental Studies (1985) *Outer Estates in Britain: East Middlesbrough Case Study*, CES Paper 26, London: Centre for Environmental Studies.
Crenson, M.A. (1971) *The Un-Politics of Air Pollution: A Study of Non- Decision Making in the Cities*, Baltimore, Md.: John Hopkins University Press.
Dake, K. (1992) 'Myths of nature: culture and the social construction of risk', *Journal of Social Issues* 48, 4: 21–37.
De Waal, A. (1989) *Famine That Kills: Darfur, Sudan, 1984–1985*, Oxford: Clarendon Press.
Douglas, M. (1985) *Risk Acceptability According to the Social Sciences*, London: Routledge.
Hance, B.J., Chess, C., and Sandman, P., (1989) 'Setting a context for explaining risk', *Risk Analysis* 9, 1: 113–17.
Hayes, M.V. (1992) 'On the epistemology of risk: language, logic and social science', *Social Science and Medicine* 35, 4: 401–7.
Hudson, R. (1990) 'Trying to revive an infant Hercules: the rise and fall of local authority modernization policies on Teesside', in Harloe, M., Pickvance, C., and Urry, J., eds, *Place, Policy and Politics: Do Localities Matter?*, London: Unwin Hyman.
Irwin, A., and Wynne, B., eds (forthcoming) *Misunderstanding Science: Making Sense of Science and Technology within Everyday Life*, Cambridge: Cambridge University Press.
Lancet, (1992) 'Environmental pollution: it kills trees, but does it kill people?', *The Lancet* 340: 821–2.
Levine, A. (1982) *Love Canal: Science, Politics and People*, Lexington, Ky: Lexington Books.
Lippmann, M., and Lioy, P.J. (1985) 'Critical issues in air pollution epidemiology', *Environmental Health Perspectives* 62: 243–58.
Lloyd, O.L. (1978) 'Respiratory cancer clustering associated with localised industrial air pollution', *The Lancet* 1: 318–20.
Lloyd, O.L., Smith, G., Lloyd, M.M., Holland, Y., and Gailey, F. (1985a) 'Raised mortality from lung cancer and high sex ratios of births associated with industrial pollution', *British Journal of Industrial Medicine* 42: 475–80.
Lloyd, O.L., Williams, F., and Gailey, F. (1985b) 'Is the Armadale epidemic over? Air pollution and mortality from lung cancer and other diseases, 1961–82', *British Journal of Industrial Medicine* 42: 815–23.
Nash, J., and Kirsch, M. (1986) 'Polychlorinated biphenyls in the electrical machinery industry: an ethnological study of community action and corporate responsibility', *Social Science and Medicine* 23, 2: 131–8.
Paigen, B., (1982) 'Controversy at Love Canal: the ethical dimension of scientific conflict', *The Hasting Center Report* 12, 2: 29–37.

Phillimore, P. (1993) 'How do places shape health? Rethinking locality and lifestyle in north-east England', in Platt, S., Thomas, H., Scott, S. and Williams, G. eds, *Locating Health: Sociological and Historical Explorations*, Aldershot: Avebury.

Phillimore, P., and Morris, D. (1991) 'Discrepant legacies: premature mortality in two industrial towns', *Social Science and Medicine* 33, 2: 139–52.

Sadler, D. (1990) 'The social foundations of planning and the power of capital: Teesside in historical context', *Environment and Planning D: Society & Space* 8: 323–38.

Scott, S., Williams, G., Platt, S., and Thomas, H., eds (1992) *Private Risks and Public Dangers*, Aldershot: Avebury.

Scott, W. (1988) 'Competing paradigms in the assessment of latent disorders: the case of Agent Orange', *Social Problems* 35, 2: 145–60.

Townsend, P., Phillimore, P., and Beattie, A. (1988) *Health and Deprivation: Inequality and the North*, London: Routledge.

Turner, B.S. (1992) *Regulating Bodies: Essays in Medical Sociology*, London: Routledge.

Part IV

Researching outcomes in health and social care

Chapter 9

Assessing health and social outcomes

Andrew Long

INTRODUCTION

Interest in measuring health outcomes has a long history, closely related to concerns over the quality of (hospital) care (Rosser 1988). Florence Nightingale introduced a daily 'outcome synopsis' of relieved/unrelieved/dead. The American surgeon Codman from the Massachusetts General Hospital suggested in 1910 that all patients should be recalled after one year to see if their treatment had achieved its initial objective. Codman's concluding question, 'What happens to the patient?', is still relevant to current practice.

A clinical concern with the outcome and quality of treatment is not unexpected, though one might question the extent to which patient perspectives are taken into account. What is perhaps more unusual is the current intense policy-level interest in outcomes. Indeed, the organization and planning of health and other public-sector delivery in the UK has long been dominated by concerns other than the evaluation of health services outcomes (Pollitt and Harrison 1992; Long 1985). For example, in 1983 a set of performance indicators (PIs) was introduced into the National Health Service (NHS) to help to assess service efficiency (Department of Health and Social Security 1983). The predominant focus lay on resource input, cost and the process of care, with only five indicators relating to outcome (Smith 1990). Few managers made extensive use of them, and where they did it was either to identify problem areas or to provide supporting evidence for policy decisions (Jenkins *et al.* 1988). At the same time, the notion of 'avoidable' deaths (Charlton *et al.* 1983; Charlton *et al.* 1986) was proposed and subsequently incorporated into the PIs, despite their accounting for a very small proportion of all deaths.

The outcome of an episode of care or health and social intervention must be related to its objectives. Defining objectives plays a key role within the cycle of strategic management – and in a strategic model these may be stated as ideal outcomes (Tutt *et al.* 1992). Clear specification of objectives is also critical within any exploration of the effectiveness of a service or programme evaluation (Holland 1983; Long 1985). Within health care, such objectives would be defined in terms of changes in health status or quality of life, and ideally based on a review of need from both professional and lay perspectives. The objective of health care can thus be described as being 'to optimize health outcomes' (Schwartz and Lurie 1990: 333).

OUTCOMES AS A POLICY CONCERN

At least five sets of policy-level concerns and initiatives can be identified within the UK context that have both pushed outcome to the centre of attention and in themselves demand an attention to outcome.

Cost containment

Pressures to contain cost have been at the heart of many policy initiatives. There has been growing pressure on all health care systems to contain costs while at the same time providing care and cure to an ageing population and keeping abreast of the development and deployment of expensive medical technologies. Relman (1988) has depicted the emphasis on patient outcome as the third revolution in medical care, providing a rational basis for improving effectiveness and efficiency and interrelating cost containment with quality improvement.

The rhetoric of the last ten years or so has been dominated by calls for value for money, efficiency in the sense of cost minimization, an emphasis on the accountability of public services, and performance review. Associated with the issue of costs is the question of the return on the investment in health and social care services. 'Outcomes are important as they form the basis of decision-making, and hence resource allocation' (Calman 1992: 29).

Effectiveness, appropriateness and variations in clinical practice

While there is research evidence of the efficacy of some treatments (a minority), questions remain about their effectiveness in the conditions of standard practice. To assess effectiveness a statement and measure of the desired, ideal and achieved outcome is required. Significant variations in clinical practice have also been uncovered (Wennberg *et al.* 1987; Wennberg 1989; Coulter *et al.* 1993). Furthermore, clinical practice may deviate from expert guidelines drawn up from research and from consensus conferences (Schwartz and Lurie 1990). Finally, health inequalities are maintained or extended, raising questions about the appropriateness of the interventions provided.

To assist purchasers the National Health Service Management Executive (NHSME) of the Department of Health (DoH) commissioned a series of Effective Health Care Bulletins (Long and Sheldon 1992) based on a systematic review and synthesis of available evidence and aimed at providing managers, clinicians and policy-makers with accessible information on the efficacy of selected medical interventions. Subjects covered so far include population-based screening for osteoporosis, rehabilitation after stroke, the management of sub-fertility, the treatment of depression in primary care, and cholesterol screening.

The promotion of quality assurance and audit

Outcomes play an important part in clinical practice, as a basis for audit and clinical research. Indeed, they are vital to standard setting and monitoring. Information on the outcome of an episode of care or treatment is in large part in the hands of the doctor. The development and promulgation of medical audit (more broadly multi-professional clinical audit – Department of Health 1993a) has thus been essential (Royal College of Physicians 1989; Hopkins 1991), though it has predominantly focused on the process of care provided to patients. But the absence of structural elements or of the failure to adhere to certain process standards does not ensure the quality of care (Schwartz and Lurie 1990; Long 1992); the link to outcome is not clearcut. Metcalfe (1990: 94) argues that clinicians need valid and reliable outcome measures 'as everyday tools of the trade'. He continues: 'as clinical audit becomes established as a mainstream activity, rather than an interest of a minority, we must make sure that process criteria . . . are justified by measurable improvements in outcome'. One notable example is the North of England Study of standards and performance in general practice (North of England Study 1992a, b).

The introduction of the internal market

The 1989 White Paper *Working for Patients*, resulting in the purchaser–provider split from 1 April 1991, introduced an explicit element of competition into the health service arena. The NHS and Community Care Act 1991 extended this to social services. Another recent addition is the Patients' Charter (Department of Health 1991a). The NHS reforms have also provided impetus to the need to put the Research and Development (R&D) function on a more secure basis and one that is more closely linked to the needs and priorities of the NHS (Peckham 1991; Hunter and Long 1993).

District health authorities (DHAs), in their purchasing role, are involved *inter alia* in the process of health needs assessment, in defining quality standards in contracts, and in developing their ability to monitor service provision, and in particular health (care) outcomes. It is important that DHAs construct a population profile that allows health status to be examined over time (Jenkins 1990). At the same time, they need to be more responsive to the needs and preferences of local people (National Health Service Management Executive 1992), involving the community in the different stages of the purchasing process. Purchasers require information not only on the costs of services, but also on the effectiveness and associated health outcomes of particular interventions, in order to decide what to purchase, in what quantity and where, and what not to purchase.

The development of a health strategy

The publication of the discussion paper (Department of Health 1991b) and the subsequent White Paper *The Health of the Nation* (Department of Health 1992) added further impetus to a focus on health outcome. It set out the government's proposals for the development of a health (as opposed to a health care) strategy for England, with the broad aim of 'improving the span of healthy life', identifying five key areas – coronary heart disease and stroke, cancers, mental illness, HIV/AIDS and sexual health, and accidents – while recognizing the need to look across the five areas in relation to the needs of specific groups of the population, for example, children and the elderly. The concept of health gain came firmly on to the policy-making and purchaser agenda. The White Paper emphasized the necessity of developing a better understanding of the clinical and cost effectiveness of interventions and the ways in which changes in health are measured. Outcome measurement 'shows not only change, but relates that change to identifiable actions, resources and events .... [and] allows the effectiveness of policies to be evaluated' with health objectives, 'not in terms of process but of improvements in health' (Department of Health 1992: 43).

The DoH discussion paper was predated by as much as two years by the work of the Welsh Health Planning Forum (1989). This outlined a statement of strategic intent for the NHS 'to take the people of Wales into the 21st century with a level of health on course to compare with the best in Europe' (ibid.: 13). The strategy set out long-term intentions, suggesting approaches for change and involving the (virtually) irreversible allocation of resources. Its foundation lay within Health for All 2000, as its guiding slogan indicated: adding years to life, and life to years. In the purchaser context, contracts would be to achieve health gain. To assist this, protocols for investment in health gain were commissioned within ten areas, including cancer (Welsh Health Planning Forum 1990) and cardiovascular disease (Welsh Health Planning Forum 1991). An agenda for action (Welsh Office 1991, 1993) outlined future priorities in terms of better quality and outcomes and their inclusion in contracts, and indicators of health gain by health-gain area as a means of tracking progress in achieving the strategic intent and direction.

At its widest level, the development of a national health strategy reinforces attention on outcome, in the particular (public health) form of health gain. It acts as a reminder that attention must lie with outcomes both for the patient and for the wider population. As part of this strategy the DoH established in 1993 a Central Health Outcomes Unit to help shift the focus of health and health care policy-making, planning, delivery and monitoring from structure and process to their effect on the health of the population served – that is, the health outcome.

A fundamental problem has been a lack of communication between clinicians, managers, planners and researchers, even when working on similar or identical problems. This results in duplication of effort, inefficient use of resources, and gaps in knowledge. The consequent lack of structured information about existing measures and techniques makes it very difficult for individuals and organizations to identify work that is relevant to their particular area, frequently resulting in the use of inappropriate measures. The development and utilization of health outcome measures remains disparate, and results frequently cannot be generalized beyond their immediate contexts. It was against this background that the NHSME of the DoH commissioned in 1992 a UK Clearing House for information on the assessment of health outcomes (Long *et al.* 1992). This provides a national resource centre of outcomes assessment material, acts as an information and advisory point and as a focal point for the exchange of information on health outcome activity, and provides critical reviews and appraisals of outcome methods and measures.

A major step for an effective outcome programme must be to enlist the commitment of the full range of decision-makers, managers and clinicians, purchasers and providers, and patients to an outcomes agenda, accepting that they may have different goals and purposes. Purchasers want to choose between provider units in terms of cost and quality, including outcome; providers also need to address effectiveness and outcomes as a way of ensuring high professional performance and to maintain contracts; and patients have always had an important personal stake in outcomes, if little voice.

This raises a crucial question about who will collect data on health services outcomes. As part of the contracting process, purchasers may specify required data (and have to pay for its collection). Changes on the R&D side (Department of Health 1993b) are also placing audit monies in their hands from 1994, raising the possibility of purchasers and providers sharing information from audit, the joint development of guidelines, and standard-setting and outcome-data requirements. Providers, independently to retain a competitive edge, will need to collect outcomes data, as part of clinical audit (as it adopts an outcome focus) and to provide evidence on quality of care and patient satisfaction to prospective purchasers. In relation to longer-term patient outcome, primary health care practitioners will have a key role to play. The establishment of effective working relationships, across the primary and secondary level, and purchasers and providers, will be critical (Frater and Costain 1992).

DEFINING OUTCOME

Although outcomes are high on the policy-making agenda, progress towards measuring and using outcomes will not be straightforward. Despite the ultimate goal of health services to improve the health of patients, it is still difficult to measure health outcomes. Indeed, there is no agreed taxonomy. This is partly due to an underdeveloped theoretical framework and a paucity of people equipped to develop, apply and interpret outcomes measures. It is thus appropriate to stand back and explore how outcomes can be defined (Long *et al.* 1993).

Outcomes, in general, are the results (effects) of processes. They are the logical consequences of an action or lack of action. They are that part of the output of a process which can be attributed to a process. The issue of attribution is often overlooked, with the measurer assuming that a process is responsible for all its outputs. An outcome of a research study might then be the study's findings or their incorporation into policy and practice. An outcome of a health or social care intervention could be improved health, successful transfer to the community, maintenance of independent living, or the patient's death. Further, it may sometimes be necessary – for example, in policy discussions to justify allocations to the health budget – to separate out and to clarify the contribution of health and/or social care services to health itself.

Health outcomes are the effects on health of any type of process. NHS and private health care services will obviously have health outcomes, but so will other areas such as housing, social services and employment. Social outcomes can be similarly defined, in particular representing the effects of such processes as housing, social services and social support.

Health services outcomes are the effects of health services. Mostly these will have effects on health, but they also include patients' satisfaction with and attitude to the services. Thus, Donabedian (1988: 178) argues that a (health care) outcome is 'not simply a measure of health, well-being or any other state. Rather it is a change in status confidently attributable to antecedent care.' Metcalfe (1990: 93) echoes this, defining outcome as 'the change in health status that results from medical (and other) interventions, or the deliberate decision not to intervene'.

It is evident that attention may be on the outcome for an individual or for the local community or a wider population. A clinician and an individual patient will be interested in the outcome of a particular intervention, which may have an effect not only on the patient, but also on the family and the community (Calman 1992). At a purchasing and public health level, interest will be in addition on the aggregate outcome of the service or intervention for the population, that is, its impact. This is mirrored in the policy-making level concern with health gain.

While there is no implicit valuation of good or bad within the concept of outcome, merely recognition of an end state, within the context of health and social care there is an expectation that the outcome of an intervention will result in a benefit to the patient or client, or at least the avoidance of a deterioration in circumstances. But who is to provide such a valuation? The perspectives of a wide range of groups need to be considered: for example, consumers, GPs, social workers, clinicians, other health and social care practitioners in the primary- and secondary-care field, purchasers, provider managers, researchers and policy-makers. Their respective interests in outcomes, and outcome measurement, may be very different. For example, consumers may be interested in outcomes in order to choose among possible treatments or to ensure that they are offered the most effective (and thus the most beneficial). Outcomes information may then empower the individual consumer. For the general public, concern may be with value for money and equity (of access and outcome). For the individual health and social care practitioner, the emphasis is likely to be on individual outcomes and on demonstrating the effectiveness of their interventions, by contrast to purchasers, who have to encompass a population perspective.

In essence, there is no single interest or reason for interest in health and social outcomes. Most importantly, the various reasons for measurement (adopting a lay and/or professional perspective) may be in competition, and the consequences contradictory. For example, the best outcome for an individual patient may compete with the notion of equity in a context of rationing (Hunter 1993).

Traditionally, health outcome measurement has concentrated on mortality and related issues such as rates of avoidable mortality. There is now an increasing concern with morbidity and health-related quality of life. Indeed Bowling (1991: 1) comments that 'measures of health status need to take both concepts (the medical model and a patient's ill-health) into account. What matters in the 20th century is how the patient feels, rather than how doctors think they ought to feel on the basis of clinical measurement.' But what is meant by health and ill-health? In its 1946 constitution the World Health Organization proposed a wide-ranging definition – a complete state of physical, mental and social well-being, and not merely the absence of disease and infirmity. However, such an ideal is not without problems, especially in any attempts to translate it into a theoretical and measurement reality (Seedhouse 1986). If this definition were to guide discussion, a health outcome would encompass a 'social', an 'economic' (for example, fitness for work) and a 'mental' dimension.

Changes in clinical indicators (cholesterol and hypertension) and risk-indicator status (smoking and exercise) are also outcomes, perceived by the patient, clinician and policy-maker to have beneficial effects. In the context of a longer-term programme concerned with the reduction of heart attack, they are not 'final' but 'intermediate' outcomes. Similarly, patient/client satisfaction with health or social care, through part of the broader assessment of the quality of the service provided, may also be perceived as an intermediate outcome (e.g. non-compliance with treatment) closely related to and influencing the final outcome (Bond and Thomas 1992; Wilkin *et al.* 1992; Carr-Hill 1992).

The range of possible health and social care outcome measures thus contains measures of the quantity of life, health-related quality of life and patient/client satisfaction. In addition, there are what might be termed 'process-based' outcome measures such as complication rates, readmission and relapse rates, which have both organizational and patient-based (intermediate) consequences (and thus outcomes). In practice, what actually gets measured will largely depend on who wants the data and for what. The critical factor is who sets the measurement agenda – clinicians, managers, researchers, patients, or some combination of these or other groups.

It is thus evident that an outcome of health and social care is more than an end-point; it involves a valuation of that end-point, and in particular a benefit to the patient/consumer. In measuring outcomes, it is thus necessary to take account of the multiple perspectives of health and social outcome; this must be reflected in the range of measures used. Further, the issue of attribution is central to the notion of outcome. Finally, there is a need to decide on an appropriate timescale in which it is reasonable to expect to see a benefit from an intervention or episode of care. In the short term the patient may improve, gaining relief from the intervention, but in the longer term may deteriorate. The optimum point for measurement from a provider's perspective may, then, be when the patient's health shows the largest improvement. Finally, there is the additional complication that if focus is on longer-term outcome, the problem of attribution becomes even more acute; many other possible causes of any observed change in health and social status may have occurred.

REVIEWING MEASURES OF OUTCOME

A wide range of instruments has been used for health outcome measurement (see Appendix). These measures (excluding mortality) aim to provide insight in a systematic and standardized way into subjective aspects of health. The opinion of the health professional and/or the patient may be sought, the latter through either an interview or a postal questionnaire. In general, the instruments consist of a set of closed questions, allow limited numbers of responses and are then translated into some form of rating to allow statistical analysis (Donovan *et al.* 1993). A minority ask patients about areas of functioning that they feel are important to their (health-related) quality of life (O'Boyle *et al.* 1992).

It is important to note that, with the exception of patient satisfaction, none as such are health outcome measures. Rather, they all represent health status instruments, and thus can be used to assess health care needs or health status at any point in time. By contrast, a health (social) outcome measure must be defined and interpreted as a measure used in the context of a health (social) (care) intervention with a view to assessing its effect. There is thus an explicit reference to it as a health (social) status instrument, but one contextualized within the assessment of the effect of an intervention. The notion of attribution is fundamental.

These measures are tools to describe and identify the end-point achieved by particular users of the process in question. They provide potentially valuable data to be used in a broader context, for example, for assessing the effectiveness and appropriateness of a health or social care intervention, or decision-making over what services to commission or to provide. The aim is to identify an instrument that is: reliable and valid; appropriate to the population or study setting; brief, easy and inexpensive to administer; and clinically credible and easily interpreted by clinicians, patients and policy-makers (Schwartz and Lurie 1990). As the previous discussion has indicated, one measure may be more appropriate for one group of users than another, and thus insufficient on its own given the diverse range of interests in health and social outcomes.

An increasing number of general and condition-specific texts are available to assist potential users to choose which of the available measures might be the most suitable instrument in their particular field (McDowell and Newell 1987; Fallowfield 1990; Bowling 1991; Wilkin, *et al.* 1992; Wade 1992; Pynsent *et al.* 1993; Swash and Wilden forthcoming). The UK Clearing House on Health Outcomes is also playing an important role here, providing advice on outcome measures and putting users of a measure, or those interested in applications in a particular area or condition, in touch with other users. Given the large number of available measures, potential users should review available measures before developing their own. 'Too often intending researchers develop their own measures, rather than embark on a systematic review of already developed instruments to find one suitable for the purpose in hand' (Wilkin *et al.* 1992: 1–2).

The instruments reviewed in the above volumes go beyond previous attempts at measuring outcome through the use of mortality data or a focus on avoidable mortality or other input–output approaches (Roberts 1990). At the same time, attempts are ongoing to use available health-services data to generate further proxy indicators of outcome (e.g. Jenkins 1990 in mental health; Milne and Clarke 1990 on the use of readmission rates; and Welsh Health Planning Forum 1991 in health-gain areas). In particular, the DoH has identified sixty or so indicators which address the outcomes area, and a working-party of the Faculty of Public Health Medicine has explored twenty of these in detail (McColl and Gulliford 1993; Department of Health 1993c). Review criteria for a health outcome measure ought at least to include consideration of the following.

CRITERIA FOR A HEALTH OUTCOME MEASURE

Conceptual basis and purpose of the measure

This includes consideration of the history and circumstances surrounding the development of the measure, and of any underlying theory of health or patient satisfaction. For example, the Sickness Impact Profile (the original American version of the Functional Limitations Profile) developed from the observation that the aim of health care is to reduce sickness, that is, the individual's own experience of illness as perceived through its effects on daily activities, feelings and attitudes. The SF-36 has its roots within cost containment and the Medical Outcomes Study (Tarlov *et al.* 1989; Stewart and Ware 1992), while the Quality Adjusted Life Years (QALY) approach (and EuroQol) seeks to address the issue of resource allocation. As Donovan *et al.* (1993: 160) comment, 'structured health status instruments largely reflect the values of their originators.'

Potential users must then query whether the purpose of the method is appropriate for their intended use. Such information may also assist in the issue of attribution, in the sense that it may be clearer how the intervention will affect the chosen outcome (measure). Indeed, as is outlined in the next section, choice of which outcome measure to employ will be determined at least in part by the theory linking the intervention to the desired or expected outcome.

Validity of the measure

The validity of a measure refers to whether or not it measures that which is intended. As this issue is well covered in standard texts (McDowell and Newell 1987; Streiner and Norman 1990), only a number of general comments will be made. First, the instrument must measure health (social) status according to some widely accepted definition. This is by no means unproblematic given the complexity of the concept of health. Second, the measure must have face validity, that is, it must cover the intended topic area clearly and unambiguously with questions related to what one wants to measure. Third, it must be determined how well the instrument works as compared with other established measures (criterion validity). Ideally, the contrast would be with some absolute 'gold standard', but this is generally unavailable (Cox *et al.* 1992). Commonly, a new instrument is compared with an established one (the SF-36 with the Nottingham Health Profile (NHP) – Brazier *et al.* 1992) or with another, shorter or otherwise more convenient instrument (Ware and Sherbourne 1992). Fourth, there is the question of how well the measure predicts future health events (predictive validity). However, this may be problematic when the measure itself is used to assist in identifying individuals at high risk and selectively treating them, and thus altering the predicted outcome (McDowell and Newell 1987). Finally, construct validity may be assessed, exploring the extent to which a particular measure relates to other measures in a way that is consistent with theoretically derived hypotheses based on the construct being measured (McHorney *et al.* 1993).

One valuable test a potential user of a measure should undertake before using it is to complete the intended instrument oneself and with colleagues, while at the same time asking and noting down reactions to the questions asked, any difficulties in responding, and thus gaining insight into whether the instrument represents one's view of health (Donovan *et al.* 1993, concerning the NHP).

Reliability of the measure

It is important to establish inter-rater reliability, repeatability (test–retest reliability) and internal consistency. McDowell and Newell (1987) point out that different uses of the measure highlight the importance of different aspects of reliability. For example, if the index is to be used to predict health outcome, then it must be able to predict itself (the test–retest criterion). If it is intended as a measure of current status, then internal consistency is more important. It must also be remembered that greater reliability implies greater validity. Cox *et al.* (1992) also observe that high inter-rater reliability may be reported for a particular measure owing to the intensive training of the interviewers, thus raising questions about its generality to the conditions of everyday practice.

Responsiveness (sensitivity) of the measure

Responsiveness can be thought of as a form of validity (Hays and Hadorn 1992). Since outcome measurement is concerned with measuring change, there is no point in using an instrument which is insensitive to clinically significant changes in an application area (Kirshner and Guyatt 1985; Guyatt *et al.* 1987). The responsiveness of a measure will depend at least on the definition of the end-point, the number of items used to cover the range and the spacing of items within this range. 'Floor' and 'ceiling' effects typically occur when an instrument designed for the general population is used in another context, such as with the severely ill, and vice versa. The NHP provides an example (Brazier *et al.* 1992), although its devisers are clear that it addresses distress rather than generic health. With multidimensional health profiles in general, interest may lie on the responsiveness of particular dimensions, depending on the application setting.

Given the original development of available measures as health-status measures, it is perhaps not so surprising that this area has been far less studied than validity; but before such instruments can be used in the context of health outcome measurement, considerable further work needs to be undertaken (Wilkin *et al.* 1992).

Degree of generalization

Cox *et al.* (1992) draw attention to the need to consider the use of the instrument in a new context. Care must be taken to test its measurement properties within the new area of application. This is particular acute with multidimensional health profiles, where the user may in fact only be interested in one or two of the dimensions of the profile. By contrast, tests of validity and reliability have been done on the instrument as a whole across dimensions.

Applicability and interpretability

Together with the above, more pragmatic issues must be considered: such as the ease of administration of the measure, its meaningfulness to the respondent and its ease of completion, as well as the broad issue of the applicability of the instrument to the particular study setting and study question. There is also the issue of the interpretability of the scores arising. To be of use in practice, they need to be easily interpreted and not to be based on complex and potentially unintelligible scoring systems. Valid interpretation will also depend on taking account of possible confounding variables (such as illness severity, co-morbidity and case mix) and issues of data quality.

It is essential that a potential user of a measure has a clear model of what is to be measured and why. In particular, this must identify what is to be measured, how the information arising will be used, and how other factors affecting the intervention can be controlled. Choice of measure needs to be informed by key criteria such as reliability, validity, responsiveness and ease of completion. It is evident that particular measures become 'fashionable' and are used almost indiscriminately, leading to an apparent consensus on their validity and reliability:

> The NHP has replaced the SIP in much research work in this way because it is perceived to be 'better' or more sensitive, but, more likely, because it is in common use. The SF-36 is now, in turn, replacing the NHP . . . . [But] issues of face validity . . . are no better resolved for this instrument than for its predecessors.
>
> (Donovan *et al.* 1993: 161)

If this is happening within research circles, how much more problematic the situation must be (and is!) in the context of discussions and applications over routine health outcome assessment within the health sector.

For an outcome measure to be used in practice its information value (informativeness) to the health practitioner and the patient/consumer must be high. There is no sense in collecting data if there is no interest in their use. At a technical level, continued attention must be given to the testing of (new) instruments and of the publication of clear descriptions of such testing and the data arising within such tests, following the recommendations of McDowell and Newell (1987). Finally, there is no single best measure; indeed, it may be the case that there is a need to use more than one, for example, a generic and a condition-specific measure (Garratt *et al.* 1993).

ASSESSING HEALTH AND SOCIAL OUTCOME

The primary concern in assessing health and social outcomes is to establish whether (process) X causes (outcome) Y under specified/controlled conditions – what Donabedian (1980) calls 'causal validity' or efficacy. In the context of multiple causation of health and illness, knowing a valid causal linkage exists only signifies the possibility of achieving a particular outcome in the conditions of routine practice. In any particular situation the outcome could have occurred for other reasons. The patient could improve spontaneously, or have been lax in adherence to the prescribed treatment, or have poor social support. Thus, can the outcome be attributed to the care in any particular situation?

To develop outcomes-assessment work, an appropriate model is required to indicate how the intervention might lead to changes in health and social status. An explicit theoretical and evidence-based model should be developed which plausibly indicates how a particular intervention can lead to the desired outcome. The approach of causal pathways (Battista and Fletcher 1988) or the 'evidence model' (Woolf 1991) can be used. The latter graphically indicates how a (clinical) outcome can be achieved, and is based on the natural history of the disease process, the sequence of intermediate effects an intervention must pass through to achieve the desired outcome, and the range of side effects that may occur. To this may be added intervening variables that may modify the link between the intervention and the outcome.

Some examples may serve to illustrate the approach. First, Fallowfield (1990) shows the links between the psycho-social problems of cancer patients – provoked by their knowledge of having a life-threatening disease and having to cope with treatment – the possible consequences of depression and anxiety, and a decline in the quality of life. Second, the notion of causal pathways is used to highlight the type of evidence that must be examined in order to evaluate the effectiveness and acceptability of an intervention within the production of the Effective Health Care Bulletins (Long and Sheldon 1992). Third, Parker *et al.* (1991) adopt a clear conceptual framework approach in their development of a multidimensional measure of outcome in child care. Starting from the proposition that the ultimate basis for child-care interventions is 'the adequate fulfilment of parental responsibilities', they explore seven dimensions for assessment: health, education, emotional development and behaviour, social family and peer relationships, self-care and competence, identity, and social presentation. These multiple dimensions provide a reminder of the problem of attribution, and thus multifactorial explanation; 'even the simplest outcome (in child care services) is shaped by forces that are either unconnected with the service or that lie largely outside its power to control' (ibid.: 28) Again, in the context of community-based care, Davies *et al.* (1990) adopt a 'production of welfare' approach in their study of the elderly and the disabled. Finally, it is the absence of an analytical model that forms a key component of the criticism made by Carr-Hill *et al.* (1987) of the approach of avoidable mortality and its potential as a valid outcome-indicator of health care. They also point to the fact that at least in this context cause and effect may be separated by years, which compounds the difficulty of attribution.

Many possible confounding variables need to be considered in any such model, and thus in any direct assessment of health outcomes. Schwartz and Lurie (1990) point to the need to adjust for case-mix, in particular the severity of the condition, co-morbidity and baseline functional status. Furthermore, 'it is difficult to derive clinically meaningful, valid, and generalisable information from patients over a prolonged period of time across multiple providers and co-morbid conditions' (ibid.: 335). The multitude of influences on patient outcome and recovery must not be overlooked: for example, patient psychology, motivation, adherence to therapy, socio-economic status, social support networks, and individual cultural beliefs and behaviour.

As the time-period extends, many other factors can intervene to modify the expected desired outcome. With multiple providers – for example, GPs, consultants, other members of the clinical teams, and patient transfers within health care and across to social care – the more difficult it becomes to attribute the outcome to one or another provider, and to disentangle the effects of one or another. Indeed, in the context of developing a seamless service (for the elderly and mentally ill, for example) it might well be counter-productive to do so. Instead, there is a need to assess multiple outcomes at a variety of times in the intervention. For example, Metcalfe (1990) suggests discharge or attendance at a follow-up clinic as easy and sensible end-points at which to assess the outcome of in-patient care. But, he continues: 'Prudence dictates as long an interval as possible . . . in order to give the maximum time for benefit to accrue . . . . The longer the measurement is left, however, the more vulnerable is the connection between intervention and outcome to intervening variables' (ibid.: 97).

A further issue is that of separating out the contribution of the various health and social care professionals to the desired outcome. Here again, a theoretical model based on research and practice is highly valuable. For example, Bond and Thomas (1991) argue for the need to establish the relationship between antecedent processes and outcomes, making explicit the intended effects and outcomes of nursing care, and encouraging the examination of unintended or unanticipated outcomes.

The major challenge is to assess health and social outcomes as part of everyday routine clinical practice. Table 9.1 outlines a possible approach. The starting-point must be the clarification of the objectives of the intervention, stated in terms of meeting health and social needs and the intended outcomes, and based if possible on research evidence of effectiveness. A theoretical model must be clarified, outlining how the intervention can lead to the desired outcome. Such a model will assist in deciding on the time dimension. Further, it will help in the choice of an appropriate health outcome measure. At another level, models of good practice need to be identified, then widely disseminated and embedded in the organization.

The most powerful method to infer causality, the randomized controlled trial, is not viable as an approach except in the context of

Table 9.1 A guide to assessing health outcomes

1 Identify objectives for the intervention, stated in terms of meeting health and social needs and the intended outcome for the patient/population.
2 Outline a theory/model to account for the expected relationship between the chosen intervention and the desired outcome.
3 Decide on the time dimension. Consider the issue of whether attention will centre on short- and/or longer-term outcome assessment. For there to be an assessment of outcome, there must ideally be a minimum of two data points, a baseline and an end-point assessment.
4 Select appropriate measures of health outcome, taking into account issues such as reliability, validity, responsiveness, ease of data collection, interpretability and informativeness.
5 Collect information on other intervening (confounding) variables, as indicated in the theoretical model, with a view to attributing the observed outcome to the intervention undertaken.

research. In order to clarify attribution, at a minimum before-and-after measurement and a comparison group (who do not receive the intervention) are required. The feasibility of such an approach within everyday health and social care practice must be queried. While imaginative research designs are needed to explore the issue of attribution (e.g. *Lancet* 1992; North of England Study 1992a, 1992b), research and development need to move closer together on the lines of health services (systems) research, with its emphasis on action-orientated and priority problem-solving undertaken in a participatory manner with decision-makers, health professionals and patients/users (Brownlee 1986; Hunter and Long 1993). Health practitioners could with value adopt the stance of the reflective practitioner (Schon 1983) and/or the (teacher) practitioner-as-researcher, and thus extend their own commitment and involvement in research as part of practice, rather than research separated from practice.

Assessing health and social care outcomes in a research study or as part of everyday practice is no easy task. As the above discussion has shown, attempts must be made to move beyond studies of efficacy to studies of outcome and effectiveness within the standard health (social) care delivery system while preserving validity and reliability (Schwartz and Lurie 1990; Gornick, *et al.* 1991). An essential first step is for health practitioners – managers, clinicians and other health and social care professionals – to accept the necessity of assessing outcomes, not just from within their own disciplinary and professional perspective but also embracing the consumer's view. An outcomes audit could be instituted, working with clinicians to develop acceptable definitions and measures of outcomes, to collect agreed outcome data, to monitor the results and to identify areas for change (Bardsley and Cole 1991).

CONCLUSION

In order to undertake effective purchasing, whether for health or for health care, purchasers must use evidence on efficacy and effectiveness to choose what (not) to purchase, on achieved outcomes to choose where to purchase, and on both effectiveness and outcomes to specify quality requirements. To choose between providers (which achieves better outcomes), outcomes data may be in the form of mortality, mobility scores, functional improvement, readmission rates, patient satisfaction, and so on. The use of such data will by no means be unproblematic. Issues of case mix, available staff mix, condition severity, social and home circumstances, and so on, will confound the interpretation. The danger lies in the uninformed use of such data, such as in the emerging league tables on provider performance. The future lies in purchasers and providers working together to produce agreed treatment protocols, including appropriate outcome indicators. Where there are gaps in knowledge, further research may be commissioned.

Health outcome measurement is fraught with methodological pitfalls, many of which need to be anticipated in planning the data collection. The enormous variety of outcome measurement requires an equally wide range of measurement strategies and designs, based on accepted methodological standards. Adopting an outcomes perspective is not just a question of choosing an appropriate measure or set of measures. It involves a long-term commitment to evaluation and audit. Furthermore, measuring outcomes is not just a matter of data collection. It requires careful consideration of why outcomes are to be assessed, an equally careful search for appropriate measures to do so, and choice of a suitable study design such that the outcome can be attributed to the intervention.

Given the wide range of outcome measures, choices will depend on the purposes in hand. A breadth in perspective must be adopted, embracing both the consumer and the professional view. It may well be the case that more than one measure is required, especially if a serious attempt is made to address the diverse reasons for interest in outcomes. This will especially be the case in the context of exploring individual and population health outcomes.

The health outcomes field is understandably preoccupied with technical concerns over reliability, validity and responsiveness and the issue of attribution, but this must not be at the expense of encouraging practitioners to measure health and social outcome and to identify the benefit of the care they are providing. It is essential to move beyond the bio-medical model, with its focus on the individual, and to acknowledge and take into explicit account the contribution of factors beyond health and social care services to health (see Chapter 10 below).

Evidence on effectiveness and outcomes and an emphasis on health gain and health outcome provide an apparently value-neutral, rational approach and means for rationing health and social care. Beneath the range of technical issues in assessing outcomes are political and social values that need to be explicit. The long-term agenda must, however, revolve around clarifying whether and how a particular intervention leads to an improvement in health or avoids a deterioration, with a view to action to improve the services provided to the individual and the population.

APPENDIX: INSTRUMENTS OF OUTCOME MEASUREMENT

1 Measures of mortality

Measures of mortality are widely used in outcome measurement, though they are increasingly supplemented by related measures of avoidable deaths and of deaths in hospitals. Their relative significance is declining as changing patterns of disease and treatment put more emphasis on measuring forms of morbidity for which mortality is not an adequate proxy.

2 Functional status measures

Some of the oldest measures come under this heading. They are designed to monitor levels of disablement or handicap as they affect the performance of basic activities such as feeding, dressing and bathing, and are sometimes known as Indices of Activities of Daily Living or even Measures of Mobility. They have mainly been developed for use in institutional settings, but more recent versions (sometimes called Measures of Instrumental Aspects of Daily Living) cover tasks more associated with living in the community, such as shopping and cooking. The Barthel index is one of the oldest and best known of the traditional measures.

3 Measures of mental health and mental illness

There are many measures of mental health, mostly concerning depression. They are often well established, widely validated and theoretically based. For outcome measurement the choice is narrowed because many of the best-known and simplest to use, such as the General Health Questionnaire and Zung Self-Rating Depression scale, are fundamentally screening instruments and not suitable for monitoring changes due to interventions. Those with necessary responsiveness, such as the Montgomery–Asberg Depression Rating Scale, tend to be difficult or expensive to administer, requiring a specially trained interviewer and taking up to an hour to administer.

4 Measures of social adjustment

Measures of social adjustment are closely related to measures of mental health. They attempt to record the extent of feeling at home in the local community and the ability to cope with immediate social surroundings.

5 Measures of social support

While the previous group of instruments explores individuals perceptions of their social surroundings, measures of social support record the links between individuals, their families and communities. They measure the level and quality of contact with friends and relatives and often include questions on memberships of community organizations such as clubs, societies and churches.

6 Measures of pain

A wide range of measures is available for measuring both pain in general, and pain associated with specific, often chronic, conditions.

7 Measures of perceived health

These instruments ask about health with questions such as: 'Would you say that your health is . . .?', or 'In the past month has your health worried or concerned you?' They aim to treat health as a unitary concept as defined by the informant.

8 Multidimensional health-status profiles

Multidimensional health status, or generic health, profiles represent a relatively recent approach to health-status measurement. They cover several dimensions of health which have previously been measured using separate instruments. At a minimum, they are likely to include items on physical functioning, role functioning, mental-health perceptions and pain. In the profile form, scores are presented for each of these dimensions, and users are generally advised against trying to combine these into a global score. The NHP (the Nottingham Health Profile) and the SF-36 (the Medical Outcomes Study 36 item Short Form Questionnaire), and the FLP (Functional Limitations Profile) are three of the best known.

9 Multidimensional health-status indices

Whereas a profile retains separate dimensions for each of its dimensions of health, multidimensional indices aim to compress this information to a single number. Indices will typically rate individual health on a scale of 1 (full health) to 0 (death), with negative values for some states of high disability and distress. The Rosser Disability/Distress scale and the Quality of Well-being Scale are two well-known examples. The more recent EuroQol contains the potential to be used as a multidimensional index, through its use of the health thermometer.

The approach can be extended by multiplying quality-of-life values by life-expectancy data for different condition groups to produce estimates of Quality Adjusted Life Years (QALY). These have been proposed as a general unit of currency for comparing the benefits of different treatments to different patient groups and therefore a rational and equitable basis for allocating resources in proportion to the measured benefits. The merits of this overall approach to decision-making and to measuring health, and the particular models used to obtain valuations, have all been hotly debated.

10 Disease-specific measures

Many clinical measuring instruments belong under this heading, as well as broader measures of health designed to be used with particular groups of patients. The Arthritis Impact Measurement Scale (AIMS) is a well-known disease-specific measure. It exemplifies the trend for disease-specific measures to cover as many dimensions of health as the general health profiles. But one must query whether it is reasonable to expect a single instrument to provide disease-specific detail on a wide range of dimensions of health. For example, can it separate depression due to arthritis from that due to other causes? And does the attention to disease-specific elements mean that the more general sections of the instrument may not have been as extensively and thoroughly developed and tested as those in the multidimensional health profiles? In the future it is possible this type of disease-specific measure will be displaced by modular packages combining a general health profile with a complementary disease-specific element. The SF-36 is already undergoing this sort of development.

11 Patient satisfaction measures

Most of the data collected concerns the patient's reaction to existing services and therefore falls far short of the kind of proactive consultation implied by some models of patient empowerment. Surveys using structured questionnaires such as the CASPE/Bloomsbury questionnaire are only one means of gaining customer feedback and have often been criticized for eliciting standardized replies. In-depth qualitative interviews such as North West Thames's Critical Incident Technique, have a higher unit cost per interview, but even a very small sample may provide a wide range of information and highlight key problems more effectively than a similarly priced large-sample survey. Other methods, such as patient advocates and more regular management contact with patients, may also provide economical and effective forms of feedback.

REFERENCES

Bardsley, M., and Cole, J. (1991) 'Measured steps to outcomes', *Health Services Journal* 17 October: 18–20.

Battista, R.N., and Fletcher, S.W. (1988) 'Making recommendations on preventive practices: methodological issues', in Battista, R.N., and Lawrence, R.S., eds (1988) *Implementing Preventive Services*, New York: Oxford University Press.

Bond, S., and Thomas, L.H. (1992) 'Measuring patients' satisfaction with nursing care', *Journal of Advanced Nursing* 17: 52–63.

—— (1991) 'Issues in measuring outcomes of nursing', *Journal of Advanced Nursing* 16: 1492–1502.

Bowling, A. (1991) *Measuring Health: A Review of Quality of Life Measurement Scales*, Milton Keynes: Open University Press.

Brazier, J.E., Harper, R., Jones, N.M.B., O'Cathain, A., Thomas, K.J., Usherwood, T., and Westlake, L. (1992) 'Validating the SF-36 health survey

questionnaire: new outcome measure for primary care', *British Medical Journal* 305: 160–4.
Brownlee, A.T. (1986) 'Applied research as a problem-solving tool: strengthening the interface between health management and research', *Journal of Health Administration Education* 4, 1: 31–44.
Calman, K.C. (1992) 'Quality: a view from the centre', *Quality in Health Care* 1: Supplement, S28–S33.
Carr-Hill, R.A. (1992) 'The measurement of patient satisfaction', *Journal of Public Health Medicine* 14, 3: 236–49.
Carr-Hill, R.A., Hardman, G.F., and Russell, I.T. (1987), 'Variations in avoidable mortality and variations in health care resources', *The Lancet* 332: 789–92.
Charlton, J.R.H., Silver, R., Hartley, R.M., and Holland, W.W. (1983) 'Geographical variations in mortality from conditions amenable to medical interventions in England and Wales', *The Lancet* 328: 691–6.
Charlton, J.R.H., Lakhani, A., and Aristidou, M. (1986) 'How have avoidable deaths indices for England and Wales changed, 1974–8 compared with 1978–83?', *Community Medicine* 8: 304–14.
Coutler, A., Klassen, A., McKenzie, I.Z., and McPherson, K. (1993) 'Diagnostic dilation and curettage: is it used appropriately?', *British Medical Journal* 306: 236–9.
Cox, D.R., Fitzpatrick, R., Fletcher, A.E., Gore, S.M., Spiegelhalter, D.J., and Jones, D.R. (1992) 'Quality-of-life assessment: can we keep it simple?', *Journal of the Royal Statistical Society* 155, 3: 353–91.
Davies, B., Bebbington, A., and Charnley, H. (1990) *Resources, Needs and Outcomes in Community-Based Care*, Aldershot: Avebury.
Department of Health (1991a) *The Patients' Charter*, London: HMSO.
—— (1991b) *The Health of the Nation*, London: HMSO.
—— (1991c) *On the State of the Public Health 1990*, London: HMSO.
—— (1992) *The Health of the Nation*, London: HMSO.
—— (1993a) *Clinical Audit Meeting and Improving Standards in Healthcare*, London: National Health Service Management Executive.
—— (1993b) *Research for Health*, London: HMSO.
—— (1993c) *Population Health Indicators for the NHS 1993, England: A Consultation Document*, London: HMSO.
Department of Health and Social Security (1983) *Performance Indicators: National Summary for 1981*, London: HMSO.
Donabedian A (1980) *The Definition of Quality and Approaches to its Assessment*, Michigan: Health Administration Press.
—— (1988) 'Quality assessment and assurance: unity of purpose, diversity of means', *Inquiry* 25: 173–92.
Donovan, J.L., Frankel, S.J., and Eyles, J.D. (1993) 'Assessing the need for health status measures', *Journal of Epidemiology and Community Health* 47: 158–62.
Fallowfield, L. (1990) *The Quality of Life: The Missing Measurement in Health Care*, London: Souvenir Press.
Frater, A. (1992) 'Health outcomes: a challenge to the status quo', *Quality in Health Care* 1: 87–8.
Frater, A., and Costain, D. (1992) 'Any better? Outcome measures in medical audit', *British Medical Journal* 304: 519–20.

Garratt, A.M., MacDonald, L.M., Ruta, D.A., Russell, I.T., Buckingham, J.K., and Krukowski, Z.H. (1993) 'Towards measurement of outcome for patients with varicose veins', *Quality in Health Care* 2: 5–10.

Geigle, R., and Jones, S.B. (1990) 'Outcomes measurement: a report from the front', *Inquiry* 27: 1–13.

Gornick, M., Lubitz, J., and Riley, G. (1991) 'U.S. initiatives and approaches to outcomes and effectiveness research', *Health Policy* 17: 209–25.

Guyatt, G., Walter, S., and Norman, G. (1987) 'Measuring change over time: assessing the usefulness of evaluative instruments', *Journal of Chronic Disease* 40, 2: 171–8.

Hays, R.D., and Hadorn, D. (1992) 'Responsiveness to change: an aspect of validity, not a separate dimension', *Quality of Life Research* 1: 73–5.

Holland, W.W. (1983) *The Evaluation of Health Care*, Oxford: Oxford University of Press.

Hopkins, A. (1991) *Measuring the Quality of Medical Care*, London: Royal College of Physicians.

Hunter, D.J. (1993) *Rationing Dilemmas in Health Care*, National Association of Health Authorities and Trusts.

Hunter, D.J., and Long, A.F. (1993) 'Health research' in Sykes, W., Bulmer, M., and Schwerzel, M., eds, (1993), *Directory of Social Research Organisations in the UK 1993*, London: Mansell.

Jenkins, L., Bardsey, M., Coles, J., and Wickings, I. (1988) *How Did We Do? The Use of Performance Indicators in the National Health Service*, London: CASPE Research.

Jenkins, R. (1990) 'Towards a system of outcome indicators for mental health care', *British Journal of Psychiatry* 157: 500–14.

Kirshner, C., and Guyatt, G. (1985) 'A methodological framework for assessing health indices', *Journal of Chronic Disease* 38, 1: 27–36.

Lancet (1992) 'Cross-design synthesis: a new strategy for studying medical outcomes', *The Lancet* 340: 944.

Long, A.F. (1985) 'Effectiveness, definitions and approaches', in Long, A.F., and Harrison, S., eds (1985) *Health Services Performance Effectiveness and Efficiency*, London: Croom Helm.

—— (1992) 'Evaluating health services: from value for money to the valuing of health services', in Pollitt, C., and Harrison, S., eds (1992) *Handbook of Public Services Management*, Oxford: Blackwell, 59–71.

Long, A.F. and Sheldon, T.A. (1992) 'Enhancing effective and acceptable purchaser and provider decisions: overview and methods', *Quality in Health Care* 1, 1: 74–6.

Long, A.F., Sheldon, T.A., and Bate, L. (1992) 'Establishment of a UK clearing house for assessing health services outcomes', *Quality in Health Care* 1: 131–3.

Long, A.F., Dixon, P., Hall, R., Carr-Hill, R.A., and Sheldon, T.A. (1993) 'The outcomes agenda: contribution of the UK clearing house on health outcomes', *Quality in Health Care* 2: 24–52.

McColl, A.J. and Gulliford, M.C. (1993) *Population Health Indicators for the NHS. A Feasibility Study*, London: Faculty of Public Health Medicine.

McDowell, I., and Newell, C. (1987) *Measuring Health: A Guide to Rating Scales and Questionnaires*, Oxford: Oxford University Press.

McHorney, C.A., Ware, J.E., and Raczek, A.E. (1993) 'The MOS 36-item short-form health survey (SF-36): II: psychometric and clinical tests of validity in measuring physical and mental health constructs', *Medical Care* 31, 3: 247–63.

Metcalfe, D.H.H. (1990) 'Measurement of outcomes in general practice', in Hopkins, A., and Costain, D., eds (1990) *Measuring the Outcomes of Medical Care*, London: Royal College of Physicians.

Milne, R., and Clarke, A. (1990), 'Can readmission rates be used as an outcome indicator?', *British Medical Journal* 301: 1139–40.

National Health Service Mangement Executive (1992), 'Purchasing for health: the views of local people', EL(92)1, 10 January, London: Department of Health.

North of England Study of Standards and Performance in General Practice (1992a) 'Medical audit in general practice, I: Effects on doctors' clinical behaviour for common childhood conditions', *British Medical Journal* 304: 1480–4.

—— (1992b) 'Medical audit in general practice, II: Effects on health of patients with common childhood conditions', *British Medical Journal* 304: 1484–8.

O'Boyle, C.A., McGee, H., Hickey, A., O'Malley, K., and Joyce, C.R.B. (1992) 'Individual quality of life in patients undergoing hip replacement', *The Lancet* 339: 1088–91.

Parker, R., Ward, H., Jackson, S., Aldgate, J., and Wedge, P. eds (1991) *Looking After Children. Assessing Outcomes in Child Care*, the Report of an Independent Working Party established by the Department of Health, London: HMSO.

Peckham, M. (1991) 'Research and development for the National Health Service', *The Lancet* 338: 367–71.

Pollitt, C., and Harrison, S., eds (1992) *Handbook of Public Service Management*, Oxford: Blackwell.

Pynsent, P.B., Fairbank, J.C.T., and Carr, A., eds (1993) *Outcome Measures in Orthopaedics*, Oxford: Butterworth–Heinemann.

Relman, A.S. (1988) 'Assessment and accountability: the third revolution in medical care', *New England Journal of Medicine* 319: 1220–2.

Roberts, H. (1990) *Outcome and Performance in Health Care*, Discussion Paper 33, London: Public Finance Foundation.

Rosser, R.M. (1988) 'A history of the development of health indices', in Teeling-Smith, G., ed., *Measuring the Social Benefits of Medicine*, London: Office of Health Economics.

Royal College of Physicians (1989) *Medical Audit – A First Report: What, Why and How?*, London: Royal College of Physicians.

Schon, D. (1983) *The Reflective Practitioner*, New York: Basic Books.

Schwartz, J.S., and Lurie, N. (1990) 'Assessment of medical outcomes', *International Journal of Technology Assessment in Health Care* 6: 333–9.

Seedhouse, D. (1986) *Health: The Foundations for Achievement*, Chichester: Wiley.

Smith, P. (1990) 'The use of performance indicators in the public sector', *Journal of the Royal Statistical Society* 153: 53–72.

Stewart, A.L., and Ware, J.E., eds (1992) *Measuring Functional Well-Being: The Medical Outcomes Study Approach*, Durham, NC: Duke University Press.

Streiner, G.L., and Norman, D.R. (1990) *Health Measurement Scales: A Practical Guide to their Development and Use*, Oxford: Oxford University Press.

Swash, M., and Wilden, J., eds (in press) *Outcomes in Neurology and in Neurosurgery*, Cambridge: Cambridge University Press.

Tarlov, A.R., Ware, J.E., Greenfield, S. *et al.* (1989) 'The Medical Outcomes Study: An application of methods for monitoring the results of medical care', *Journal of the American Medical Association* 262, 7: 925–30.

Tutt, N., Neale, J., and Warbuton, W. (1992) 'Strategic management in social service', in Pollitt, C., and Harrison, S., eds (1992) *Handbook of Public Services Management*, Oxford: Blackwell.

Wade, D.T. (1992), *Measurement in Neurological Rehabilition*, Oxford: Oxford University Press.

Ware, J.E., and Sherbourne, C.D. (1992) 'The MOS 36 item short-form health survey (SF-36), 1: conceptual framework and item section', *Medical Care* 30: 473–83.

Welsh Health Planning Forum (1989) *Strategic Intent and Direction for the NHS in Wales*, Cardiff: Welsh Office NHS Directorate.

—— (1990) *Protocol for Investment in Health Gain: Cancers*, Cardiff: Welsh Office NHS Directorate.

—— (1991) *Protocol for Investment in Health Gain: Cardiovascular Diseases*, Cardiff: Welsh Office NHS Directorate.

Welsh Office (1991) *NHS Wales: Agenda for Action 1992 to 1994*, Cardiff: Welsh Office NHS Directorate.

—— (1993) *Advice on Outcomes*, 'Contracting for Health Gain' Project, Cardiff: Welsh Office NHS Directorate.

Wennberg, J.E. (1989) 'The agenda for outcomes research', in Hopkins, A., ed., *Appropriate Investigation and Treatment in Clinical Practice*, London:Royal College of Physicians.

Wennberg, J.E., Freeman, J.L., and Culp, W.J. (1987) 'Are hospital services rationed in New Haven or over-utilised in Boston?', *The Lancet*, 332: 1185–9.

White, A., Nicholass, G., Foster, K., Browne, F., and Carey, S. (1993) *Health Survey for England 1991*, Office of Population Censuses and Surveys, Social Survey Division, Series HS no. 1, London: HMSO.

Wilkin, D., Hallam, L., and Doggett, M.A. (1992) *Measures of Need and Outcome for Primary Health Care*, Oxford: Oxford University Press.

Woolf, S.H. (1991) *Interim Manual for Clinical Practice Guideline Development: A Protocol for Expert Panels Convened by the Office of the Forum for Quality and Effectiveness in Health Care*, Washington, DC: US Department of Health and Human Services, Agency for Health Care Policy and Research.

Chapter 10

Health needs assessment, chronic illness and the social sciences

Ray Fitzpatrick

INTRODUCTION

The assessment of need is an essential step in the selection of appropriate therapy for an individual patient. It has now become a public health priority in the determination of the health services required to serve populations (Department of Health 1989). A fundamental part of the public-health physician's training and working 'tool-kit' has always been epidemiology, and expectations are high that this discipline will play a fundamental role in health needs assessment. However, delineating the incidence and prevalence of the various chronic illnesses, difficult enough as a task by itself, is not the same as identifying needs for health care. Chronic illnesses pose a powerful challenge to epidemiological logic because, for any particular illness, there is enormous variation between individuals in the nature and severity of health problems, and also considerable change in the nature of problems over time and in the degree of benefits obtained from health care interventions.

The social sciences have made many distinctive contributions to our understanding of chronic illnesses, emphasizing in particular the importance of the sufferer's own perspective regarding his or her illness (Blaxter 1976; Anderson and Bury 1988). Such work has a vital function in sensitizing health professionals and others to the experiences of the chronically ill, but it has yet to have an impact on clinical and managerial decision-making in health services.

However, most recently, a 'revolution' has been acclaimed which is intended to enable the insights of the social sciences (particularly regarding the experience of chronic illness) to be integrated into population- and practice-based information systems, resource-allocation mechanisms and, above all, clinical decision-making of health care systems (Ellwood 1988; Relman 1988). This revolution is the enhanced ability that now exists to use information systems for the first time to measure and monitor the outcomes of medical interventions: 'The centrepiece and unifying ingredient of outcomes management is the tracking and measurement of function and well-being or quality of life' (Relman 1988: 1552). This paper is a critical review of the revolution, particularly as it relates to health needs assessment for the chronically ill.

THE DEVELOPMENT OF ASSESSMENT TECHNIQUES

At the heart of the revolution is the development by social scientists in collaboration with epidemiologists and clinicians of a vast array of survey-based instruments. These take the form of questionnaires or interview schedules to assess what is now variously referred to as the patient's 'quality of life', 'functional status', 'health profile', 'subjective health status' or simply 'health status'. They have in common that they are intended as practical, economical, reliable and valid means of obtaining aspects of patients' personal experience of symptoms and the associated physical, social and psychological sequelae of their illness. Some of the instruments have been developed to provide assessments of the various consequences for health status of specific diseases, for example, breast cancer (Levine *et al.* 1988) or rheumatoid arthritis (Meenan *et al.* 1980). However, another tradition has emphasized the development and use of generic instruments that might be applicable to a wide range of health problems, most notably instruments such as the Sickness Impact Profile (Bergner *et al.* 1981) and the Nottingham Health Profile (Hunt *et al.* 1985). This array of instruments offers potential insights relevant to health needs assessment.

Richer information

The first and most obvious attraction of these health status measures is that they provide richer and more specific information about subjects than do more conventional assessments. Many of the early standardized clinical assessments (e.g. the Karnofsky Performance Index (Karnofsky and Burchenal 1949)) operated within unidimensional scales of function, well-being or disability, thereby failing to allow for independence between dimensions (for example, the possibility of individuals with poor mobility but excellent psychological well-being). In addition, many such scales operated with small numbers of categories that distinguished only gross differences between patients. Most of the new instruments provide a more detailed and differentiated description of respondents.

Ability to distinguish between patient groups

Health status instruments can distinguish between groups with different kinds of health problems, such as individuals with different chronic illnesses (Stewart *et al.* 1989), and draw attention to particular health problems of social groups such as the socially deprived or unemployed (Ahmad *et al.* 1989).

Predictive of demands upon health services

Health status instruments have now been widely applied to the various predictive tasks required in health care systems. They have been shown to predict patterns of health service use, long-term morbidity, mortality, and volume and costs of out-patient and in-patient care (Pincus *et al.* 1984; Wolfe *et al.* 1988).

Improving health professionals' awareness of health problems

There is fairly extensive evidence that health professionals are not sensitive to the personal and social consequences of chronic illness amongst their patients. Doctors may be unaware of a substantial amount of the disability in their patients (Calkins *et al.* 1991). They may underestimate morbidity (Fossa *et al.* 1990) and misjudge patients' views of their quality of life (Slevin *et al.* 1988). They may underestimate the consequences for personal and family life of chronic illnesses (Cooper and Huitson 1986). The potential role of health status instruments in clinical care is therefore substantial and would include practice- and attender-screening to identify cases and use of instruments as an aid to individual patient care and to monitor progress of care (Nelson *et al.* 1990).

Assessment of outcome in clinical trials and health service evaluation

The role of health status measures in the assessment of the outcomes of health care is a crucial application of such instruments. A review of the issues regarding outcomes assessment is beyond the scope of this discussion. An aspect of outcomes research that is relevant to health needs assessment is provision to patients of outcomes information based on prior research, to promote more shared decision-making between patient and health professional (Wennberg 1990).

Thus it would appear that the scope for applying health status instruments in health needs assessment is extensive. However, there remain a number of fundamental issues to be resolved before we can accept that a revolution has occurred with regard to health needs assessment for the chronically ill. We have first to determine the extent to which new methods can claim to capture salient aspects of health problems from the patient's perspective. Second, we have to consider what kinds of health needs assessment are actually feasible.

Sensitivity to salient aspects of chronic illness

One of the most valuable features of the more recent health status instruments is that they are multidimensional, i.e. they distinguish different aspects of illness experience, such as physical function, pain, emotional consequences, social consequences which cannot be reduced to a single dimension. In the field of rheumatology the most established instrument – the Arthritis Impact Measurement Scales (AIMS) – distinguishes between nine aspects of health status that need to be assessed in individuals with rheumatoid arthritis: mobility, physical activity, dexterity, household activities, activities of daily living, social activity, anxiety, depression and pain (Meenan *et al.* 1980). Not only has the instrument been shown to have basic measurement properties of reliability, acceptability and construct validity; it has also been shown to be sensitive to improvements in health status brought about by several different drugs (Anderson *et al.* 1989). Yet when some patients with rheumatoid arthritis were asked to complete a different instrument – the Notttingham Health Profile (NHP) (Hunt *et al.* 1985) – one of the dimensions with the worst scores for patients, and with scores most distinct from 'normative' population scores was 'energy', i.e. feelings of tiredness and loss of energy (Fitzpatrick *et al.* 1992). Feelings of fatigue are quite characteristic in patients with rheumatoid arthritis and are a salient aspect of the experience of the disease (Tack 1990). The fact that this aspect of illness experience should be omitted from the 'state of the art' and most established of health status instruments should signal caution against the unthinking assumption that 'validated' instruments will necessarily fit the bill for all possible requirements.

Even where different instruments do appear to cover similar dimensions and therefore appear to be equivalent for the purposes of assessment, this may be illusory. Thus, for example, most instruments now include at least one scale that assesses the 'social dimension' of health status. This dimension was explored in relation to the different pictures of patients with rheumatoid arthritis that were presented by two established health status instruments (Fitzpatrick *et al.* 1991b). A sample of hospital patients completed both the AIMS and the NHP on two occasions three months apart. Whereas for dimensions such as mobility and emotional aspects, the two instruments produced consistent scores, for the social scale, whether cross-sectionally or expressed as change over time, individuals' scores on the two instruments hardly agreed at all. From other data gathered, as well as from inspection of the content of the social scales of the two instruments, it was clear that they covered different phenomena. While the NHP was concerned with more perceptual and emotional aspects of individuals' relations with others (such as 'feeling a burden'), the AIMS instrument is more concerned with behavioural and structural aspects of individuals' social networks (such as frequency of contact). There is substantial evidence that these are generally two quite distinct aspects of individuals' social relationships (Seeman and Berkman 1988). The two health status instruments appear to be tapping two important but different phenomena. One needs to be clear-minded in determining aspects of health status relevant to the matter at hand and in selecting the most appropriate measures.

Detecting change

Another technical problem that has only recently begun to be addressed is the sensitivity to change of such instruments. Many chronic illnesses are characterized by short-term as well as long-term fluctuations in the severity and nature of symptoms. In a study of disability in south London (Patrick and Peach, 1989), 70 per cent of the disabled respondents experienced a significant degree of change in their disability over a two-year period. The issue of whether instruments are sensitive to such changes is absolutely crucial when they are used as 'before-and-after' scores to assess the benefits of treatment. Instruments that may have substantial validity in terms of differentiating between individuals at a point in time may well have very poor sensitivity to changes within individuals over time (Guyatt *et al.* 1987). In the case of chronic illnesses with substantial inherent variation over time, the problems associated with detecting beneficial (or indeed harmful) effects of health care interventions become particularly acute.

These problems can be illustrated from a sample of patients with rheumatoid arthritis who, by their own judgement and by a variety of clinical and laboratory data, had experienced some significant improvement over a three-month period. The extent to which these improvements were reflected in the changes in scores for four health status instruments completed by patients at the beginning and end of the three-month period was examined (Table 10.1). We are not here concerned with how accurate the instruments really were in measuring change, since there is no final court of appeal to address such a question. The point of the table is to illustrate the argument that the picture of the degree of change experienced by these patients varies according to one's choice of health status instrument. For example, mobility changes appeared modest according to the NHP and substantial according to the Functional Limitations Profile (FLP) (Patrick and Peach 1989). Again, pain would appear to have been substantially improved according to AIMS but only moderately improved according to the NHP. At the most extreme, no improvements occurred according to the social dimension of AIMS, whereas the corresponding scale of the FLP detected quite substantial improvements.

One of the most important considerations that still requires serious examination is the extent of serious omissions amongst the new arrays of instruments. Many different aspects of the experience of chronic illness highlighted by recent social scientific work on chronic illness are not yet incorporated into health status instruments. Thus, for many conditions a sense of uncertainty is a central feature of the experience of illness (Fitzpatrick *et al.* 1993). In other conditions, the stigma and sense of differentness is marked (Scambler 1989). Other studies emphasize the importance of a sense of control over symptoms (Fitzpatrick *et al.* 1990), desires to understand the purposes of treatments (Jobling 1988) or the need to maintain a sense of normality regarding identity (Kelleher 1988). Such experiences are salient features of chronic illness that should be incorporated into health status assessments.

FEASIBLE CONTRIBUTIONS TO HEALTH NEEDS ASSESSMENT

Prevalence surveys

There are therefore a number of technical and conceptual issues still to be addressed in assessing health status. In addition, it is important to consider strategic questions as to how health needs assessment of the chronically sick may be facilitated by the availability of health status instruments. One obvious application is to supplement conventional descriptive epidemiology. Health status instruments have a role in

Table 10.1 Degree of change indicated by four different health status instruments*

Dimension	*Effect Size* **
Mobility	
AIMS	*0.43*
HAQ	*0.38*
NHP	*0.27*
FLP	*0.69*
ADL	
AIMS	*0.26*
HAQ	*0.28*
FLP	*0.46*
Household	
AIMS	*0.38*
HAQ	*0.74*
FLP	*0.26*
Pain	
AIMS	*0.73*
HAQ	*0.53*
NHP	*0.38*
Mood/Emotions	
AIMS	*0.83*
NHP	*0.59*
FLP	*0.61*
Social	
AIMS	*0.06*
NHP	*0.24*
FLP	*0.60*

ADS = Activities of Daily Living; AIMS = Arthritis Impact Measurement Scales; HAQ = Health Assessment Questionnaire; NHP = Nottingham Health Profile; FLP = Functional Limitations Profile

* From a sample of patients with rheumatoid arthritis considered to have improved over a three-month period.
** Effect size = difference between mean score at time 1 and mean score at time 2, divided by standard deviation at time 1. Effect size of 0.20 or less considered small, 0.50 moderate, and 0.80, or higher, large (Kazis *et al.* 1989).

providing information about the prevalence of perceived health problems and social consequences of chronic illness in the local population or general practice list (Curtis 1987). Such surveys may draw attention, for example, to the poorer scores across many dimensions of health status experienced by individuals with mental illness (Wells *et al.* 1989) or to the distinct and different problems experienced by individuals with different chronic illnesses (Stewart *et al.* 1989). In this sense, such evidence has a sensitizing or publicizing function in graphically drawing attention to local health problems of concern to public health medicine.

However, much of this local use of health-survey instruments by public health medicine has been described provocatively as 'displacement activity that is professionally reassuring at a time of uncertainty, rather than as a productive means of "health needs assessment"' (Frankel 1991: 258). Health status instruments in population surveys may well draw attention to the health needs of one geographical area or social group relative to another within a population (Ahmad *et al.* 1989). However, it may well prove to be the case that such evidence of the relative health needs of one group compared with another can be obtained more economically from more readily available health data such as deprivation indices (Morris and Carstairs 1991).

The general problem with subjective health status information obtained from population surveys is that it inevitably remains somewhat broad and non-specific. Few, if any, instruments to date assess the level of subjective demand for health care in relation to subjective health status. Thus, problems identified in population surveys have an uncertain relation to levels of felt need for health care. Similarly, from the health care provider's perspective, subjective health status problems are insufficiently specific to identify levels of medically determined need for particular health care interventions. In this respect, health status instruments may yet prove as disappointing as conventional epidemiological methods, which all tend to be stronger in measuring the prevalence of particular pathological phenomena than in identifying the extent of need for particular health care interventions (Frankel 1991).

This is not to argue against all forms of health status measurement in population surveys. We still do not have sufficient population-based information about levels of disability and other health problems in relation to specific chronic diseases. Such surveys, in addition to health status information, need to obtain clinically relevant data to obtain standardized diagnoses and evidence of capacity to benefit from medical interventions (Frankel 1991). Such work is expensive and long-term, but still needs to be done. Reservations are about the value of routine use of instruments in the more immediate tasks of needs assessment in local public health medicine.

Population targets

A more feasible application of health status instruments on a population basis may be in setting targets. The government has adopted as a core principle of its broad strategy for health the setting of specific targets (Secretary of State for Health 1991), a principle fully supported by the Faculty of Public Health Medicine (1991). It is hoped that specific targets will serve to clarify objectives, mobilize activity, and facilitate evaluation efforts over time.

Many chronic illnesses might well be neglected by strategies based upon targets, for the basic reason that targets require an ability to measure progress. For many health problems, mortality is an appropriate measure, and relevant targets that command assent can be identified with relative ease. The burden of ill-health imposed by, for example, rheumatoid arthritis is not captured by mortality statistics, and such diseases may therefore risk being omitted from the logic of targets. Health status instruments or the constructs and dimensions which they highlight may provide an invaluable inspiration for the development of targets for chronic illness. Does the social-scientific and epidemiological literature on chronic illness point to possible targets that could command assent?

In rheumatology a very simple self-completed questionnaire was developed – the Health Assessment Questionnaire (HAQ) – which has a number of valuable properties (Fries *et al.* 1980). It is short (twenty items), and is known to be reliable and to have satisfactory construct validity (Brown *et al.* 1984). It assesses a core set of constructs, mainly ability to perform a number of everyday tasks. From the perspective of targets, the problems which it measures are intrinsically and incontestably undesirable, so that value judgements about quality of life are not a salient issue. The instrument has been shown to be responsive to health care interventions (Wolfe and Cathey 1991a). However, it is now clear that it would warrant consideration as a target for other reasons. It is highly predictive of long-term functional loss and mortality (Wolfe and Cathey 1991b). Thus, an instrument like the HAQ has a number of advantages as a source for targets. It also has limitations. The predictive power of the instrument has been established largely in clinic populations known to be clinically homogeneous from other information. It is not clear how well such instruments would perform in the more uncertain environment of a population survey. Above all, it is disease-specific and unlikely to be of general use, for example in chronic illnesses where upper-limb function is less affected.

Another example might be the setting of targets with regard to social integration. The Faculty of Public Health Medicine advocates the following targets in relation to individuals with physical disability: (a) the proportion of people with a physical disability who belong to a social or recreational group should not differ from the proportion in the general population; (b) 95 per cent of people with a physical disability should speak to a friend or relative at least once a week and feel that there is at least one person who cares about them. The advantage of such targets is not only that they are simple and capable of being monitored. Of equal importance is the now substantial evidence that social integration is an important predictor of well-being in chronic illness (Patrick and Peach 1989; Fitzpatrick *et al.* 1991a). There is still research to be done to identify more precisely optimal and economic measures of social integration. However, we have the basis for targets that might be incorporated into a regular disability survey, in Office of Population Censuses and Surveys style. Overall, the difference between this use of health status instruments compared with applications in prevalence studies is one of purpose and practicality. In this application, one is using evidence about the social consequences of chronic illness selectively to focus on particular issues to be prioritized in a fairly pragmatic way. The prevalence study to examine health status and social consequences of chronic illness, because of its more wide-embracing scale and scope, has to be used more sparingly to address more scientific questions.

At a national and international level, quality of life and disability are increasingly of interest to incorporate into targets such as 'expectation of life without disability' (Bebbington 1988) and 'healthy life expectancy' (Robine and Ritchie 1991). Fries (1989) continues to argue that the scope for 'compression of morbidity' is extensive and that indicators such as disability-free life years should therefore be a central part of national health strategies. The importance of different diseases as targets also shifts if such concepts are measured. For example, the elimination of loco-motor disorders would make a negligible contribution to increasing life expectancy, but a very substantial one to disability-free life years gained. Such data may also be used, for example, to show that inequalities of health between socio-economic groups are greater if one uses disability-free life expectancy compared with simple life expectancy (Robine and Ritchie 1991). As more sophisticated measures of disability and methods of combining disability and survival data become available, more complex expressions of the construct of healthy life expectancy will be used (Rogers *et al.* 1989).

Applications in clinical contexts

As indicated earlier, clinicians fail to observe many of the health-related problems of disability and quality of life in the patients who consult them. A number of reviews (Almy 1988; Rubenstein *et al.* 1989a) and editorials of medical journals (Wolfe and Pincus 1991) have therefore advocated the routine use of instruments to assess functional, social and psychological aspects of health status in clinical practice. These applications differ from population prevalence studies in that in this context patients have expressed a need for health care by consulting the doctor.

A number of studies have been conducted that explore the role of health status instruments in increasing clinicians' awareness of broader aspects of patients' health problems and improving their forms of management. One of the most encouraging of studies involved the use of functional-status screening to assess the frail elderly in a specialist in-patient unit of a veterans' hospital. Experimental (screened) patients showed improvements over controls in both mortality and functional outcomes (Rubenstein *et al.* 1984).

Generally studies have been less encouraging regarding the value to clinicians of health status reports about their patients. Thus, in one study (Kazis *et al.* 1990), 1920 patients with rheumatoid arthritis were assigned either to a study condition in which their doctors received quarterly results from health status instruments completed by the patient, or to one of two control groups in which results were not fed back to the doctor. There were no observable differences at the end of the year, either in terms of process measures such as referrals or medication changes, or in terms of outcome measures such as compliance, satisfaction or health status change. One possible reason for the failure to obtain benefits from feeding back health status information was that doctors had not been educated about the purpose and content of health status instruments. However, a similarly designed study of 510 experimental and control group patients receiving primary care included a two-hour education programme for the experimental group of doctors (Rubenstein *et al.* 1989b). However, again no differences were obtained in terms of either process or outcome measures.

Despite the overall disappointing results of these two randomized controlled trials, it is noteworthy that a majority of clinicians in both studies who received reports regarded the information as useful, not in informing specific clinical decisions, but in improving communication about health status or helping the doctor–patient relationship. A third study of this kind suggested that a minority of doctors felt instruments provided fresh information about the patient and improved doctor–patient communication (Nelson *et al.* 1990). Interestingly, this third study also evaluated patients' views. The vast majority liked completing the instruments; nine out of ten felt the information was important for the doctor to know, and three-quarters felt it influenced communication with their doctor. The value to the patient of such techniques has so far been relatively unexplored.

Given that clinical attitudes were broadly positive to the receipt of information about health status, it is worth considering reasons for the failure to influence processes or outcomes. The simplest explanation in the case of the two randomized trials is that information was not fed back immediately or to coincide with surgery visits by the patient. This minimized the scope for doctors to act on the information. Further explanations may be sought in the view that health status information remains inherently arcane in format and lacks clinically intuitive meaning. The obscurity of, for example, health status change scores is often cited as a barrier to wider clinical use (Deyo and Patrick 1989). Because of the view that most existing instruments remain too long and are impractical for regular clinical use, a recent trend has been to produce shorter forms of instruments. Thus the Dartmouth Primary Care Cooperative Information Project (COOP) has developed a set of nine simple pictorial 'charts' in the domains of physical, emotional, role and social function, overall health, change in health, pain, overall life quality and social support (Nelson *et al.* 1990). Instruments such as the COOP chart attempt to provide assessments across the spectrum of patients' health problems without the level of detail of other generic instruments such as the Sickness Impact Profile. Studies will therefore be needed to identify how much is lost in terms of relevant information about patients' health status in return for the gains of brevity and simplicity.

Patients' concerns

Patients who present their chronic health problems to doctors vary considerably in the nature and focus of their concerns (Fitzpatrick and Hopkins 1983; Brody and Miller 1986). Although health status instruments attempt to assess by different methods the severity of different problems, they generally have not addressed the problem that patients will differ considerably in the extent to which an aspect of disability or health-related quality of life is a concern or considered something for the doctor to address. Some recent developments begin to address this issue in ways that may make clinical applications of health status instruments more useful.

It has been suggested that, if patients selected aspects of health status or quality of life that were of particular concern to them, this would be a more appropriate base-line from which to evaluate interventions (MacKenzie *et al.* 1986). Some studies have begun to explore the use of more individualized health status instruments, in which patients select personal health status priorities, in the fields of cardiorespiratory disease (Guyatt *et al.* 1987) and patients undergoing surgery (MacKenzie *et al.* 1986).

Other evidence suggests the value of acknowledging individual differences with regard to management of their chronic illnesses. Patients have different preferences for radical vs conservative treatment for life-threatening diseases (McNeill *et al.* 1982). Patients vary in whether they expect information, reassurance and support as opposed to more active medical treatments in relation to chronic illnesses (Fitzpatrick and Hopkins 1983). Such variation between patients within categories of health problem can only be addressed by methods that elicit individual concerns and expectations.

DISSEMINATION OF OUTCOMES RESULTS

Finally it should be reiterated that one of the main areas in which health status and quality-of-life measures should play a role *vis-à-vis* chronic illness is in providing evidence of the outcomes of different procedures. Those who view outcomes research as a centre-piece of a revolution in medicine are matched by those who believe that developments are likely to be slower, more complex and less dramatic (Epstein 1990). However, there is a major contribution that outcomes evidence will eventually make to needs assessment. For both doctor and patient, more standard and patient-entered data will eventually emerge as to the different kinds of outcomes of health care intervention. This should enable both parties to make more considered and informed choices about health-care needs, based on accessible evidence about outcomes of alternatives.

CONCLUSION

It is possible to focus too exclusively on the health status or quality-of-life deficits of the individual with a chronic illness, thereby ignoring the impact that the social context has in shaping and determining handicaps. One danger of the 'revolution' that has been reviewed here is that it will reinforce the tendency to look at ways in which the individual has health-related problems requiring personal adjustment and thereby to ignore changes in the broader context which may more readily improve quality of life. Thus, for example, amongst individuals with rheumatoid arthritis, over half of those who worked before the onset of the disease may expect to lose their job within ten years of diagnosis (Yelin 1990). Although disease and disability variables explain some of the variance in work outcome, far more variance is explained by various characteristics of the job, such as degree of physical demands, and level of discretion in pacing of work activities. Thus, employment policies may well need to be the focus of interventions to improve many aspects of well-being for individuals with disabling illness. Similarly, housing and transportation policies will certainly make a crucial difference to other aspects of daily life for the chronically sick. Although outside the immediate responsibilities of health authorities, such factors are clearly not outside the public health function. The Department of Health's document *The Health of the Nation* (Department of Health 1992) explicitly recognizes the contributions of other departments and sectors in contributing to health.

However, this review has focused largely on the interface between individuals with chronic illness and the NHS. We have now an abundance of evidence concerning the diversity of experiences, concerns and problems confronted by such individuals, and increasingly there are also the means to make such concerns visible. Strategies for health continue to be limited by available data, which largely comprise mortality and health service activities. Careful consideration should now be given to the role and value of methods that get closer to illness experience. The very heterogeneity of the concerns and experiences consequent upon chronic illness revealed by such methods is our best evidence of the scope for 'compression of morbidity' in this large group of health problems.

REFERENCES

Ahmad, W., Kernohan, E., and Baker, M. (1989) 'Influence of ethnicity and unemployment on the perceived health of a sample of general practice attenders', *Community Medicine* 11: 148–56.

Almy, T. (1988) 'Comprehensive functional assessment of elderly patients', *Annals of Internal Medicine* 109: 70–2.

Anderson, R., and Bury, M. (1988) *Living with Chronic Illness*, London: Unwin Hyman.

Anderson, J., Firschein, H., and Meenan, R. (1989) 'Sensitivity of a health status measure to short-term clinical changes in arthritis', *Arthritis and Rheumatism*, 32: 844–50.

Bebbington, A. (1988) 'The expectation of life without disability in England and Wales', *Social Science and Medicine* 27: 321–6.

Bergner, M., Bobbit, R., Carter, W., and Gilson, B. (1981) 'The Sickness Impact Profile: development and final testing of a health status measure', *Medical Care* 19: 787–805.

Blaxter, M. (1976) *The Meaning of Disability*, London: Heinemann.

Brody, D., and Miller, S. (1986) 'Illness concerns and recovery from URI', *Medical Care*, 24: 742–8.

Brown, J., Kazis, L., Spitz, P., Gertman, P., Fries, J., and Meenan, R. (1984) 'The dimensions of health outcomes: a cross-validated examination of health status measures', *American Journal of Public Health* 74: 159–61.

Calkins, D., Rubenstein, L., Cleary, P., Davies, A., Jette, A., Kosecaff, J., Young, R., Brook, R., and Delbanco, T. (1991) 'Failure of physicians to recognise functional disability in ambulatory patients', *Annals of Internal Medicine*, 114: 451–3.

Cooper, G., and Huitson, A. (1986) 'An audit of the management of patients with epilepsy in thirty general practices', *Journal of the Royal College of General Practitioners*, 36: 204–11.

Curtis, S. (1987) 'Self reported morbidity in London and Manchester: inter-urban and intra-urban variations', *Social Indicators Research*, 19: 255–72.

Department of Health (1989) *Working for Patients*, London: HMSO.

—— (1992) *The Health of the Nation*, London: HMSO.

Deyo, R., and Patrick, D. (1989) 'Barriers to the use of health status measures in clinical investigation, patient care, and policy research', *Medical Care*, 27: S254–S268.

Ellwood, P. (1988) 'Shattuck Lecture – outcomes management', *New England Journal of Medicine* 318: 1549–56.

Epstein, A. (1990) 'The outcomes movement – will it get us where we want to go?', *New England Journal of Medicine* 323: 266–70.

Faculty of Public Health Medicine (1991) *The Health of the Nation: Faculty Response*, London: Faculty of Public Health Medicine.

Fitzpatrick, R., and Hopkins, A. (1983) 'Problems in the conceptual framework of patient satisfaction research', *Sociology of Health and Illness* 5: 297–311.

Fitzpatrick, R., Newman, S., Lamb, R., and Shipley, M. (1990) 'Helplessness and control in rheumatoid arthritis', *International Journal of Health Sciences* 1: 17–24.

Fitzpatrick, R., Newman, S., Archer, R., Shipley, M. (1991a) 'Social support, disability and depression: a longitudinal study of rheumatoid arthritis', *Social Science and Medicine* 33: 605–11.

Fitzpatrick, R., Ziebland, S., Jenkinson, C., Mowat, A., and Mowat, A. (1991b) 'The social dimension of health status measures in rheumatoid arthritis', *International Disability Studies* 13: 34–7.

Fitzpatrick, R., Ziebland, S., Jenkinson, C., Mowat, A., and Mowat, A. (1992) 'A generic health status instrument in the assessment of rheumatoid arthritis', *British Journal of Rheumatology* 31: 87–90.

Fitzpatrick, R., Robinson, I., and Scambler, G. (1993) 'Patient-based assessments of health status and outcome for some neurological disorders', in Molgaard, C., ed., *Epidemiology of Neurological Disorders*, San Diego, Calif.: Academic Press.

Fossa, S., Aaronson, N., Newling, D., Van Caugh, P., Denis, L., Kurtz, H., and de Pauw, M. (1990) 'Quality of life and treatment of hormone resistant metastatic prostatic cancer', *European Journal of Cancer* 26: 1133–6.

Frankel, S. (1991) 'The epidemiology of indications', *Journal of Epidemiology and Community Health* 45: 257–9.

Fries, J. (1989) 'The compression of morbidity: near or far?', *Milbank Quarterly* 67: 208–32.

Fries, J., Spitz, P., Kraines, R., Holman, H. (1980) 'Measurement of patient outcome in arthritis', *Arthritis & Rheumatism* 23: 137–45.

Guyatt, G., Walter, S., Norman, G. (1987) 'Measuring change over time: assessing the usefulness of evaluative instruments', *Journal of Chronic Diseases* 40: 171–8.

Hunt, S., McEwen, J., McKenna, S. (1985) 'Measuring health status: a new tool for clinicians and epidemiologists', *Journal of the Royal College of General Practitioners* 35: 185–8.

Jobling, R. (1988) 'The experience of psoriasis under treatment', in: Anderson, L., and Bury, M., eds., *Living with Chronic Illness*, London: Unwin Hyman.

Karnofsky, D., and Burchenal, J. (1949) 'The clinical evaluation of chemotherapeutic agents in cancer', in Macleod, C., ed., *Evaluation of Chemotherapeutic Agents*, Symposium at New York Academy of Medicine, New York: Columbia University Press.

Kazis, L., Anderson, J., and Meenan, R. (1989) 'Effect sizes for interpreting changes in health status', *Medical Care* 27: S178–S189.

Kazis, L., Callahan, L., Meenan, R., and Pincus, T.(1990) 'Health status reports in the care of patients with rheumatoid arthritis', *Journal of Clinical Epidemiology* 43: 1243–53.

Kelleher, D. (1988) *Diabetes*, London: Routledge.

Levine, M., Guyatt, G., Gent, M., DePauws, S., Goodyear, M. (1988) 'Quality of life in stage II breast cancer: an instrument for clinical trials', *Journal of Clinical Oncology* 6: 798–810.

MacKenzie, R., Charlson, M., DiGioia, D., Kelley, K. (1986) 'A patient-specific measure of change in maximal function', *Archives of Internal Medicine* 146: 1325–9.

McNeill, B., Parker, S., Sox, H., Tversky, A. (1982) 'On the elicitation of preferences for alternative therapies', *New England Journal of Medicine* 306: 1259–62.

Meenan, R., Gertman, P., and Mason, J. (1980) 'Measuring health status in arthritis: the Arthritis Impact Measurement Scales', *Arthritis & Rheumatism* 23: 146–52.

Morris, R., and Carstairs, V. (1991) 'Which deprivation? A comparison of selected deprivation indexes', *Journal of Public Health Medicine* 13: 318–26.

Nelson, E., Landgraf, J., Hays, R., Wasson, J., and Kirk, J. (1990) 'The functional status of patients: how can it be measured in physicians' offices?', *Medical Care* 28: 1111–26.

Patrick, D., and Peach, H. (1989) *Disablement in the Community*, Oxford: Oxford University Press.

Pincus, T., Callahan, L., Sale, W., Brooks, A., Payne, L., and Vaughan, W. (1984) 'Severe functional declines, work disability and increased mortality in seventy-five rheumatoid arthritis patients studied over nine years', *Arthritis & Rheumatism* 27: 864–72.

Relman, A. (1988) 'Assessment and accountability: the third revolution in medical care', *New England Journal of Medicine* 319: 1220–3.

Robine, J., and Ritchie, K. (1991) 'Healthy life expectancy: evaluation of global indicators of change in population health', *British Journal of Medicine* 302: 457–60.

Rogers, R., Rogers, A., and Belanger, A. (1989) 'Active life expectancy among the elderly in the United States: multistate life-table estimates and population projections', *Milbank Quarterly* 67: 370–411.

Rubenstein, L., Josephson, K., Wieland, G., English, P., Sayre, J., and Kane, R. (1984) 'Effectiveness of a geriatric evaluation unit: a randomised controlled trial', *New England Journal of Medicine* 311: 1664–70.

Rubenstein, L., Calkins, D., Greenfield, S., and Jette, A. (1989a) 'Health status assessment for elderly patients: report of the Society of General Internal Medicine task force on health assessment', *Journal of the American Geriatric Society* 37: 562–9.

Rubenstein, L., Calkins, D., Young, R., Cleary, P., Fink, A., Kosecoff, J., Jette, A., Davies, A., Delbancor, T., and Brook, R. (1989b) 'Improving patient function: a randomized trial of functional disability screening', *Annals of Internal Medicine 110:* 836–42.

Scambler, G. (1989) *Epilepsy*, London: Routledge.

Secretary of State for Health (1991) *The Health of the Nation*, Green Paper, London: HMSO.

Seeman, T., and Berkman, L. (1988) 'Structural characteristics of social networks and their relationship with social support in the elderly', *Social Science and Medicine* 26: 310–57.

Slevin, M., Plant, H., Lynch, D., Drinkwater, J., and Gregory, W. (1988) 'Who should measure quality of life, the doctor or the patient?' *British Journal of Cancer* 57: 109–12.

Stewart, A., Greenfield, S., Hays, R., Wells, K., Rogers, W., Berry, S., McGlynn, E., and Ware, J. (1989) 'Functional status and well-being of patients with chronic conditions', *Journal of the American Medical Association* 262: 907–13.

Tack, B. (1990) 'Fatigue in rheumatoid arthritis', *Arthritis Care Research* 3: 65–70.

Wells, K., Stewart, A., Hays, R., Burnam, A., Rogers, W., Daniels, M., Berry, S., Greenfield, S., and Ware, J. (1989) 'The functioning and well-being of depressed patients', *Journal of the American Medical Association* 262: 914–9.

Wennberg, J. (1990) 'Better policy to promote the evaluative clinical sciences', Quality *Assurance in Health Care* 2: 21–9.

Wolfe, F., and Cathey, M. (1991a) 'Analysis of methotrexate treatment effect in a longitudinal observational study: utility of cluster analysis', *Journal of Rheumatology* 18: 672–7.

Wolfe, F., and Cathey, M. (1991b) 'The assessment and prediction of functional disability in rheumatoid arthritis', *Journal of Rheumatology* 18: 1298–1306.

Wolfe, F., and Pincus, T. (1991) 'Standard self report questionnaires in routine clinical and research practice – an opportunity for patients and rheumatologists', *Journal of Rheumatology* 15: 643–6.

Wolfe, F., Kleinheksel, S., Cathey, M., Hawley, D., Spite, P., and Fries, J. (1988) 'The clinical value of the Stanford Health Assessment Questionnaire functional disability index in patients with rheumatoid arthritis', *Journal of Rheumatology* 15: 1480–8.

Yelin, E. (1990) 'Health care research and technology', *Current Opinion in Rheumatology* 2: 237–35.

Name index

Subject index

Lightning Source UK Ltd.
Milton Keynes UK
UKOW051126020212

186515UK00001B/15/A